AFFIRM
& BURN!

A fun, easy way to a lighter, healthier you!

J. OCCHIO, M.S. ED.

Because WEIGHT LOSS begins in the MIND, not in the BODY!

AFFIRM & BURN!™

Disclaimer: The information in this book may not be construed as a medical diagnosis, treatment, advice, claim, or substitute for a physician's care. Consult a physician or health care provider before starting a weight loss or exercise program. There are no promises you will be successful. Success depends on you!

Author's note: My hope is that this book will make you really want to get lighter and healthy. And it starts with no dieting or exercise. *Affirm & Burn!* will work great alone, or in combination with any diet or exercise program.

AFFIRM: To make firm or confirm; to state or assert in a positive way; to express dedication to.

They affirmed that the goal of a lighter, healthy body would be achieved.

BURN: To use up; to destroy by fire.

They visualized burning all their negative, limiting thoughts and beliefs.
They burned unwanted calories.
They "burned rubber" headed for the finish line.

AFFIRM & BURN!
WHAT IT IS AND HOW IT WORKS

Have you noticed the first question many of us ask a person who has lost weight? You guessed it: "How did you do it?" Why? I believe it is because we are all searching for an EASIER WAY to get light and healthy, and since a large percentage of us fail at this, we want to know how anyone achieves what appears to be impossible. Sure, millions of people have been able to lose weight at times during their lives, yet over 90 percent of them gain it all back. The question is, "Why?"

Is it because we have no idea what to do? I don't think so. Knowing what to do is not the difficult part. Information about what to eat and how to exercise is available just about everywhere. What it's really about is motivation, and motivation always starts in the mind.

That's what *Affirm & Burn!* is all about.

Affirm & Burn! is a remarkably simple, one-of-a-kind, totally positive, health and fitness book designed to work your mind as well as your body. It's a book designed to simply make your journey to a lighter, healthier body a more pleasurable experience.

By simply reading and "playing" with *Affirm & Burn!* over time, you will actually become a person who truly wants to eat healthy and exercise on a regular basis. This may sound a little crazy, but it's that kind of passion you want and need when it comes to your health.

The truth is, we are all a little crazy or passionate about something in some way. If you are significantly overweight, chances are you are just a little too passionate about eating too much food, and most likely, the wrong foods. The point of this program is to show you how to bring out that passion you may have for food and focus it on something you know is more important in your life: eating healthier and exercising. So why get crazy about your health and fitness program? Because getting a little crazy or passionate about something is what makes that something much easier to do.

I'll give you an example. Have you heard of the 90-something, health and exercise guru Jack LaLanne? He passed in 2011, but he was a man who had been eating healthy, exercising daily, and living a vigorous life for over 75 years. Seventy-five years! At the age of 70 he actually swam a portion of the Long Beach Harbor in California pulling 70 boats with one person in each boat. That is passion! This was a man whose mind was totally focused on health and fitness. Now, do you need to be as passionate as Jack LaLanne was? Of course not. What you do want to do, however, is conjure up a small amount of that passion so your journey to a lighter, healthier, body becomes a lot easier. Yet, how does one do that? How do you develop a passion to do something?

You do it by working with your mind and convincing yourself first that there will be so much pleasure in doing what you set out to do. This is what playing with *Affirm & Burn!* does. It teaches you how to make healthy eating and exercising pleasurable. It helps change your mindset from being one type of pleasure-seeking crazy person—the pleasure from excessive, wrongful eating and inactivity—to another type of pleasure seeking crazy person: the "health and fitness" pleasure-seeking crazy person.

The truth is that for all of us human beings, everything simply comes down to feeling good as much as you can. That is what billion-dollar food and beverage corporations associate to their products. It is also the main objective of advertising.

If you think about it, almost all food and beverage ads are saying, "If you are not feeling good, consume this and then you will feel good! *Affirm & Burn!* does the same thing, but in a much more authentic and healthy way. It will help you to affirm how much better you will feel by simply eating better foods and exercising on a more regular basis.

Feeling good is not very difficult when your body is healthy and your mind is focused on something positive. Wouldn't you agree? If you love to eat unhealthy foods because they make your mouth feel good and your body less stressed, you will eat lots of unhealthy food every day to feel good as much as you can. We all do this at times, it is just that some of us are doing too much of it and it is the main reason for being overweight. It is a feel good formula that millions of us have so easily gotten hooked on, yet is ultimately flawed.

Unhealthy foods can in fact make you feel good while you're eating them, but the weight they cause us to gain hurts us physically and psychologically for a much, much longer time. If you are overweight, you know this to be true, but you most likely don't think about the serious negative consequences. Therefore, it seems as though there is no problem, but there is, and the problem exists in the mind. The mind is so powerful and we can simply choose to put any kind of consequences out of our minds, but no matter how clever we are at doing that, we cannot put the consequences of an unhealthy lifestyle out of our body.

Ignoring serious consequences of overeating, and instead continuing to focus on the temporary pleasurable taste and perhaps calming feeling that comes over the body as all that extra food is digested, is the type of thinking that creates an unhealthy body. It's the kind of thinking that needs to change and it is not very hard to do when you read *Affirm & Burn!* and do the simple, fun mind exercises.

Affirm & Burn! will inspire you to change your present attitude (in simple ways) of choosing to live an unhealthy lifestyle, which so many mistakenly believe is pleasurable, to that of choosing to live a healthy lifestyle, which truly is pleasurable. Your attitude is so important, and is greatly affected by what you consistently say and think every day. Are you truly aware of what you often say and think about food and exercise?

Many of us believe eating healthy and exercising is a difficult, cumbersome task. Are you one of them? It absolutely does not have to be that way. Believing and thinking like that is a big part of the problem. Many of us also make it much more difficult for ourselves when we often unknowingly affirm how much we love fattening foods and being lazy. Have you ever heard someone say something like, "I loooove pizza. I loooove ice cream, cookies or pie. I can eat a bucket of French fries and fried chicken and sit on the couch every night. I hate working out. I don't have time to exercise"? These are very harmful things to say if a person's desire is to get light and healthy! Why? Because the mind will believe and obey anything you tell it. As silly as it may sound, the more a person consistently affirms unhealthy statements, especially in an emotional way, the more difficult it becomes for them to lead a healthy lifestyle. *Affirm & Burn!* is here to help change that.

Affirm & Burn! is designed to get you to think and feel extremely positive about living a healthy lifestyle so that you see it as something you really want to do instead of something you or others think you should do. It all starts with changing the way you think and what you say throughout the day. It's just that simple. You might now ask, "How will *Affirm & Burn!* change the way I think?"

Affirm & Burn! uses a variety of fun (yes, fun!), powerful techniques that affect your mind in subtle ways. You might say the methods are very similar to those used in advertising. They include the use of powerful affirmations, rhymes, and other methods to help get you very excited about doing what you know you should do. It is a series of techniques that you have most definitely experienced if you've seen television commercials, infomercials, billboards, magazine ads, newspaper ads, online pop-up ads, or any other form of advertising.

Let's face it. We're all bombarded by advertising designed to get us to do things we do not particularly want or need to do. Have you ever seen a fast food commercial, an ad in a magazine or on a huge billboard? Of course you have. Did an ad ever influence you to do something? I'm sure one has at some time. If it did not affect us, it probably affected our peers who then gradually influenced us to engage in the behavior. Advertising does in fact work in influencing us, or companies would not continue to spend billions of dollars on it.

Imagine using these same highly persuasive techniques to help make getting healthy easier. Imagine creating an environment for yourself where everything you saw, read, or heard emphasized how great it feels for you to eat healthy and exercise every day. That is a very powerful concept, and *Affirm & Burn!* is the first book to utilize it. Since advertising can't be stopped, it is time to be aware of it and use it to our advantage by customizing it to our needs.

You might say *Affirm & Burn!* is like a self-induced billion dollar healthy eating and exercising ad campaign. The purpose of the campaign is to bombard your mind and sell yourself on the incredible benefits of living a healthy lifestyle. Its job is to get you to the point where you absolutely love healthy food and exercising so much that you no longer desire junk food or being lazy. It is designed to help you create such great mental focus and enthusiasm on doing healthy, fat-reducing, exercise-oriented, things that it does not seem difficult at all. You actually enjoy it. Yes, it's true: you will actually want to eat healthy food and exercise instead of forcing yourself to do so.

Here's a question for you. If you ever tried to eat healthier or start exercising, why did you do it? Maybe a doctor, family member, or close friend suggested it, or you just decided to do it. Ultimately it was a decision you made in your MIND. After a certain amount of time, however, you stopped. Why? You simply changed your mind! A negative, uninspiring thought entered your mind and you acted on it. Perhaps you made the decision that it was "too difficult to keep eating healthy and too inconvenient to exercise." You may have also added that there was "no joy in life if you could not eat all the fattening foods you liked and had to suffer through a workout at least three times a week". You most likely convinced yourself with consistent thoughts like these that ultimately led you to believe there was constant suffering and very little pleasure in doing this, so you chose to stop. Why? It is because in your mind eating what you want and not having to exercise was always pure pleasure and very easy.

What is the bottom line here? The truth is that we all seek pure pleasure and things being easy. This is the concept *Affirm & Burn!* works with. It shows you how you can follow the simple program and convince yourself that eating healthy and exercising can be pure pleasure and easy! It does this by bombarding you with so many affirmations and other powerful techniques to convince you that pure lasting pleasure comes from eating healthy and exercising on a regular basis. And if you follow the program for several weeks, you will no longer need a lot of convincing. You will become addicted to good health habits. Your mind, body, and soul will "get it," and want to stick with this better way of life forever. Imagine that. Living a life where you naturally want to eat healthy food, exercise, and feel great all day long. You can get there, and *Affirm & Burn!* will make it fun and easy for you.

Affirm & Burn! was created by asking better questions to people that have succeeded in getting light and healthy and staying that way. And the questions were not about how they did it. The questions were "What were you thinking and saying just before you started your program? What were you thinking and saying every day during your program? What are you thinking and saying every day, now, to stay light?

When you get the answers to these most important questions, you have then found the true first step to the secret of getting light easily—and staying there easily for the rest of your life.

CHAPTER 1

SOME FREQUENTLY ASKED QUESTIONS

What do you mean by *Affirm & Burn!* using advertising techniques?

All people living in developed countries are bombarded by advertising. The advertising techniques used (in the form of beautiful and colorful images with compelling words and catchy phrases) are all designed to tap into your subconscious mind (the little kid in you), and they work. If they didn't work, companies would not spend billions of dollars on advertising! So if companies spend billions using techniques to get you to buy certain items or eat and drink things you know you should not, imagine how much more effective these techniques would be if you actually wanted to do what they were designed to make you do.

If you follow the simple instructions in *Affirm & Burn!* you will soon notice it working on you, but you must do it. Do exactly what the instructions say: be a little silly, have fun, and experiment. Think of *Affirm & Burn!* as a game to be played. Be a kid again. Play the simple game. Put your favorite affirmations where you can see and read them often, and soon you will become a believer. Read them on your phone or tablet when you wake up, before you sleep, and throughout the day. The more you do it, the more effective it will be.

So, where do you start?

The greatest thing about *Affirm & Burn!* is that it doesn't start by eliminating a person's favorite fattening foods and/or going to the gym to exercise. Most people find their mind and body are not ready for this. A person will struggle to do that because the mind perceives that as suffering. This is why very few people are able to stay on a diet for a long time, and why the few who do almost always gain the weight back. If you have not trained your mind properly, it is painful to stay on a diet when in your mind you do not want to be on one; you find it pleasurable to go off the diet and eat whatever you want. So the key is to first make everything about eating healthy and exercising a pleasurable experience and bombard the mind with that powerful message. This is the essence of the *Affirm & Burn!* philosophy. The positive, feel-good aspects of eating healthy and exercising must be consistently affirmed first in the mind, so you really want to become a lighter, healthier, happier person and stay that way because it gives you consistent pleasure.

And once again, it all starts in the mind. You must prepare and train your mind first because everything begins in thought. The mind is the ultimate source of all your power. When your mind is trained and convinced that eating healthy and exercising is going to be the greatest experience ever, it will be so much easier for you to then take action and make positive healthy changes in your life. You will do it because you really want to, not because you should or because someone else told you to. So, once again, in the beginning, there are absolutely no food restrictions or requirements to exercise until you are mentally ready for it. No suffering. Ever!

So, how will *Affirm & Burn!* first train your mind? How does it work?

The first step with *Affirm & Burn!* is to simply decide that getting light and healthy is something you absolutely want to do. That's it. No exceptions! Once you have made this simple but vital decision, *Affirm & Burn!* becomes your greatest support system in keeping you totally focused and happy on your journey to a lighter, healthier body.

Affirm & Burn! does this by showing you how to bombard your brain with large amounts of positive, empowering information. Most of this takes place in the form of simple, one-line, affirmations. These affirmations have been carefully designed to create incredibly positive focus on the benefits of eating healthy and exercising. In other words, as you read them over and over daily, with conviction, you will become a person who is motivated and knows that great lasting pleasure ultimately comes from eating healthy foods and exercising, which are the keys to getting light and healthy. (When and how to read the affirmations and do the simple exercises appears later in the book.)

After several weeks of programming your mind with the techniques of *Affirm & Burn!* and you find yourself actually wanting to eat healthy and exercise, you'll set a date for a Health Ceremony. This is simply an enjoyable personal ritual that pleases your subconscious and conscious mind and further commits you to a healthy lifestyle. It is the final, most meaningful step to easily attaining your health goal. You might compare it to a wedding ceremony.

In a wedding ceremony two people commit their lives to taking care of each other. This is exactly what you are doing with a Health Ceremony, except the relationship is between you and your body. It is the first and most important relationship you can have—the one that truly does always last "until death do you part."

Another important thing to note if you are in a committed relationship is it's always much easier to take care and get along with others when you are healthy. That's why, in many ways, your Health Ceremony is more important than a wedding ceremony. It is a ritual that demonstrates you have decided you love your body, enjoyed your body's response to healthy food and exercise, and are ready to commit to taking care of it by eating healthy and exercising for the rest of your life. A Health Ceremony is a beautiful thing and plays an important role in truly living "happily ever after" with that special someone! (The Health Ceremony is further explained later in the book.)

I'm a little afraid. Is this going to change who I am? I really love food. What if I do this and I stop loving the foods I've always loved? What if I become a crazy health nut or exercise addict?

There is absolutely nothing to be afraid of. We are all crazy whether we are light or not, and can choose to be whatever we want at any time. You are always in control with *Affirm & Burn!*. You can always go back to the old you if you choose to do so at any time. Your love of food is not about food—it's about love. *Affirm & Burn!* is simply going to help you transfer some of that love of food to a love of eating healthy and exercising. That's it! You will still love and eat food, but it will be healthier, better quality food, and not oversized amounts of it. So don't be afraid. Being afraid of this is as silly as being afraid of getting healthy when you are really sick and your body is in pain. Play with *Affirm & Burn!* for a few weeks as if it were a new toy. Give it a chance, always knowing you can choose to put all the information away and go back to your old habits if you wish.

Affirm & Burn! is designed to introduce new, empowering ideas to your conscious and subconscious mind so that living a healthy lifestyle becomes a more pleasurable experience. That's it. Getting healthy can and should be as easy and fun as possible! That's what this book is about. To better understand how this book will help you, however, let's learn more about how your conscious and subconscious mind works.

CHAPTER 2

Your Conscious and Subconscious Mind

"The mind's imagination is more powerful than knowledge."
- Albert Einstein

"He who is fixed to a star does not change his mind."
- Leonardo DaVinci

"The mind is everything. What you think, you become."
- Buddha

"There is nothing good or bad but thinking makes it so."
- Shakespeare

"Change your thoughts and you change your world."
- Norman Vincent Peale

"A man is but the product of his thoughts, what he thinks he becomes."
- Gandhi

"Most folks are about as happy as they make up their minds to be."
- Abraham Lincoln

"How did I do it? I just changed my mind."
- Anonymous

Your conscious mind is the part of your mind that centers on reason and logic. It decides what is right or wrong for you. (It is what is reading and understanding these words right now.) It acts like a parent to another more powerful part of your mind in your head called the subconscious mind.

Your subconscious mind (your inner child, the little kid in you) is separate from your conscious mind. It acts like a powerful computer that will simply run any program you put into it, good or bad. It can't make decisions like the conscious mind or even know the difference between what is true or what you think is true. It does, however, have the power to make you do things you no longer consciously wish to do, like overeating.

Why does it have this power? It's because over time, it was programmed by your consistent thoughts and actions. Your thoughts and actions were mostly a product of how you were raised, your environment, the people you spent time with, and of course your own free will. As your subconscious kept hearing all the words and thoughts about things that contributed to weight gain, it created an overweight person.

Your subconscious program is basically the sum of all the habits you have developed over the years. You know that once something becomes a habit, it's easy for you to do it. Some habits that you may have picked up might include overeating, smoking, drinking alcohol, biting your nails, drinking coffee every morning, etc.

So the subconscious simply runs the program (habits) of your life, both good and bad. Since you were born, your subconscious mind has been taking in both appropriate and inappropriate information. If you are overweight, your conscious mind (parent) has simply taught your subconscious mind (inner child, the little kid in you) improper eating habits and the habit of being physically inactive over the years. These habits then became the program of your subconscious mind and you simply ran the program. The subconscious, which, like a machine, is incapable of deciding right from wrong, simply followed your instructions. It picked up on everything, much like a recorder that records ALL noise when turned on. Whatever was said or thought, good or bad, it heard.

Over time you may have taught it the following without even realizing it:

Food tastes great, so eat as much as possible whenever you can.

Eat food to feel better when you are bored or lonely, even if you're not hungry.

Eat food when you are happy, even if you're full, and it will make you happier.

Eat food when you are sad and the sadness goes away.

Eat as much as you can to get your money's worth.

Never, ever waste food no matter how full you are.

Always finish everything on your plate even if you are full.

Exercising is not important. There is never enough time to exercise.

You can live without exercising; you can't live without food.

Eat whatever you like; you only live once.

It's not my fault I'm overweight; it's my genes.

Look around, everyone else loves to overeat and is heavy so it's OK.

I'm not as fat as her. I'm not as fat as him.

Never ever refuse extra food from a friend, relative, or client even if you are full because you might hurt their feelings.

Exercising is difficult and boring, so why do it? We are all gonna die anyway.

I'm "SICK AND TIRED" of hearing that I should eat better and exercise more.

And so on.

Can you see how difficult it would be to eat healthy and exercise if you had thoughts like that consistently running through your head, or worse, if you said those statements out loud and often? If you have often had thoughts like the ones above, your subconscious was listening very carefully and is now simply running this self-destructive weight-inducing program whether you are aware of it or not.

Again, the subconscious (the little kid in you) does not know right from wrong; it just does what it is told. That is why it is extremely important to become aware of what one is thinking and saying because the subconscious is ALWAYS listening and ready to do whatever is programmed into it. You must become aware of statements like "I'm sick and tired of," because you are telling your subconscious to welcome illness and low energy, and it will do what it is told.

Wouldn't it be interesting if you found yourself saying the opposite? Instead of saying, "I'm sick and tired of dieting and trying to lose weight," say, "I'm healthy and energized about this new *Affirm & Burn!* program that is going to get my mind right before I even try to diet or exercise again!" Try saying that every time you catch yourself about to say "sick and tired" for a few weeks, and see what happens. It's a fun experiment!

In fact, say this out loud right now. "I'm healthy and energized about this new *Affirm & Burn!* program that is going to get my mind right first so that eating healthy and getting lighter from now on will be fun and easy!"

Did it feel good to say that? Or at least a little better than "sick and tired?" Be honest. It must have!

Remember: your actions, good and bad, are executed easily and effortlessly by the program of your subconscious mind without you even being conscious of it.

The subconscious is also where your body gets its energy. That "little kid in you" has access to a bundle of energy! If you know how the kid in you thinks and what inspires him/her, you can teach him/her new tricks and tap into incredible power. That kid can help make changes in your life a whole lot easier. Your subconscious can be your greatest and most powerful friend!

Think of a time in your life when you were so excited about something that you could not sleep at night, and yet you still had enough energy for the next day. This was your subconscious letting energy flow through. The little kid in you can give you the energy to accomplish anything when you understand how to work with him/her. Remember, the kid is like a robot with a computer running a program, and a computer's program can be changed.

What exactly is your subconscious mind and how can it work for you?

Think of your subconscious (little kid in you) as a five-year-old child who is very impressionable, like a fantastic listener who hears and remembers everything and is in charge of your body. He/she is also a part of your self that communicates with you not in words, but through your body, feelings, and dreams. Unfortunately, you do not always get the message, because he/she does not speak in plain English, like those times when you are afraid or nervous in a particular situation and you consciously do not understand why. That is your subconscious trying to talk to you! He/she is saying, "Hey, I'm afraid. We've never done this," in the language of an upsetting feeling in your gut.

Then, when you reassure him/her and repeat that situation over time (conquer the fear), your subconscious eventually learns the lesson and stops creating that uncomfortable feeling. In other words, it understands and works for you instead of against you. If you only knew how much is going on inside your subconscious mind, you could fix many of your problems. However, this process takes time and everyone must work at their own comfortable pace.

The secret is paying attention to what you are saying and doing, and how it is affecting you.

How do you communicate with the subconscious mind (inner child/kid) and get it to change?

The first step is to relax the body and clear the conscious mind. This is what hypnotists do. You allow the hypnotist to relax you and he/she puts aside your conscious mind simply because you agree to let them do that. Then the hypnotist talks to your subconscious to give you a new set of beliefs that support what you wish to do. However, some people feel uncomfortable with this. They do not like the idea of being put to sleep and having another person "program" them. This is understandable. Fortunately there are other ways to affect your subconscious mind program where YOU have all the power and ability to change the way you want to change. One simple way is through the use of powerful affirmations. That is what *Affirm & Burn!* is mostly about.

OK, remember: the subconscious is also known as the inner child, age five or six. It is in kindergarten! And like most kids in kindergarten or first grade, he/she likes to play and be happy. Just like a kid, it likes hearing short fun stories that teach a simple lesson. It enjoys seeing things (visuals) it likes and wants. It likes colors too. And the more it sees things like this throughout the day, the more of a reality it becomes in life for it and you. It also likes toys, games, and winning—right now!

Picture yourself walking into a kindergarten class dressed like the current, lovable, most popular cartoon character with a huge box of the latest, treasured toys. Then you tell the kids you are going to play a game so they can win these toys. You will see some motivated kids! They will jump up and down and be ready to go. That is how you have to think in terms of motivating YOUR subconscious. That's how it will unleash its supportive energy for you and that's why this book focuses on the positive fun stuff!

It is all about working with the power of your inner child and changing your whole attitude toward eating right and exercising by working with your conscious and subconscious mind. Once all the good stuff seeps into the subconscious mind, you will be on automatic pilot and programmed for a lean healthy body. There will be no more suffering. Your healthy lifestyle of eating right and exercising will be something you naturally want to do.

That's it. Hopefully you understand a little more about what is going on with the little kid inside that skull of yours! The good news is, even if you do not understand any of this psychological stuff, it doesn't matter! Just play with *Affirm & Burn!*. It will still work on you if you play along and do the simple exercises without understanding how it works. See the whole thing as an exciting, positive experiment and have fun with it.

Eating healthy, exercising, losing weight, and keeping it off can be easy. It all starts by simply making the decision to totally commit to your health and fitness goal. After you do that, *Affirm & Burn!* is there to help make the process easier by helping you transform yourself into a person who loves healthy food and exercise.

So have fun with *Affirm & Burn!* and enjoy learning how to think and act like a lighter, healthy, happy person!

AN INTERESTING, FUN WAY OF GETTING STARTED

An interesting way to begin this program is to use your mind and its unlimited power of imagination. Albert Einstein used his unlimited power of imagination to come up with his greatest contribution to science: the theory of relativity. You can use yours as well in your approach to weight loss.

Imagine you were suddenly washed ashore to a beautiful island in the Pacific. For some reason, you could not remember how or why you got there. All you knew was that you were there with nothing but the clothes on your back, yet you were calm and optimistic. You are then suddenly greeted by a group of friendly, nonjudgmental people who treat you like a treasured old friend who had simply been away for a while. They take you to a beautiful hotel-like room that contains all of your basic necessities: a comfortable bed, bathroom, shower, toiletries, etc. A very pleasing, refreshing, fragrance suddenly fills the air of this room.

You then take a walk outside and notice the island's perfect landscape. Beautiful trees, flowers, and colorful birds inhabit this breathtaking paradise. You soon notice that all of the people on this island are happy and in fantastic shape because they think positively, eat only healthy food in proper portions, love their work, and exercise every day. You too then begin to eat, think, work, and exercise just as they do. In a short time you begin to notice yourself getting lighter and happier every day without trying. You feel like you are in a paradise—and you are. You have no interest in junk food, fast food, or being lazy, because you are naturally eating, moving, being positive, and feeling great every day.

This is the essential message of *Affirm & Burn!* It is here to help you create this "island mindset" in your own mind so that your journey to a lighter, healthier body becomes something that simply happens in a gradual, natural, enjoyable way, the same way it would happen on the island. Use the photo that follows or get a photo from a vacation booklet or the Internet and give this island a name. Make it part of your Health Ceremony if you like. Remember that you can "escape" to this island in your imagination any time you wish instead of escaping with junk food.

Let's begin!

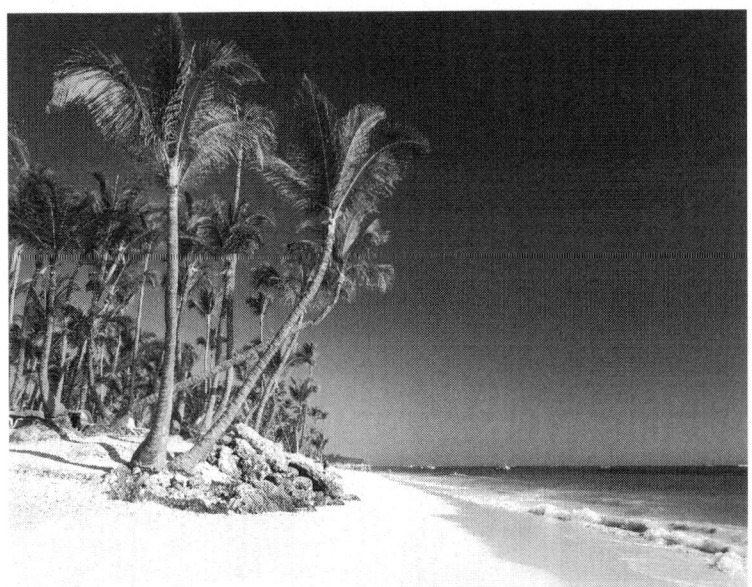

CHAPTER 3

Awesome Affirmations and Power-Rhyme Affirmations

What exactly are affirmations? Affirmations are positive statements that help you focus on what you want. They can have a profound effect on how you act and feel when you repeat them often (with feeling) and are the basis of this program.

You have thousands of thoughts each day whether you want to or not. What you think about most affects your subconscious mind (the little kid in you), expands, and ultimately becomes your reality. If your goal is to get light and healthy in an enjoyable way, the majority of your thoughts about health and fitness need to be positive and empowering.

You may have trouble at times coming up with creative ways of thinking more positively. The affirmations provided here will help you address this problem. They were created to help you focus on the many positive ways to think about eating healthy and exercising in spite of any difficulties going on in your life.

When you repeat these affirmations often, and with conviction and feeling, they will make an impression on your subconscious mind, helping you to act on and achieve your health goals more easily. They work best when you repeat often the affirmations that feel most comfortable, powerful, and truthful to YOU. Repetition with conviction is key!

A light, healthy person who enjoys eating healthy food in proper portions, as well as daily exercise, often has thoughts like the affirmations listed below. The idea is for you to adopt the same thoughts so you think and ultimately act just like a light and healthy person. Once you allow the affirmations to sink deeply into your subconscious, you will want to exercise and eat healthy foods in proper portions. It will feel natural to you, just as eating fattening foods, overeating, and being inactive may have seemed natural to you in the past.

DIRECTIONS:

1. Simply find a place where you can be calm and undisturbed for five to ten minutes.

2. Read all the affirmations, including the power rhyme affirmations, highlighting those that stand out most for you (screenshot them if you are reading this on a smart phone or tablet). You may like them all or just a few. Like songs, everyone has their favorites. What matters most is **finding the affirmations that have truth and meaning for you.** This will be your personalized list that you will enjoy reading every morning and at bedtime. (This is a mandatory but simple assignment that takes only three to five minutes, so there is no excuse not to do it!)

3. After you have completed step 1, go to your personalized list and pick out your top four affirmations (or rhymes): Choose two from the starter affirmations list, one from the eating list, and one from the exercise list.

Post the two starter affirmations in the bedroom, where you can see, read, and repeat them as soon as you wake up. Post one eating and one exercise affirmation in the bathroom—on the mirror, above or near the shower head, on the wall opposite the toilet bowl, etc., where you can repeat them out loud or in your mind as you brush your teeth or wash your face for the day. These are the two most important rooms, because no matter how busy you are, you always have a few minutes to read and repeat your affirmations in these places. The shower is an especially fun place to repeat a power-rhyme affirmation. Following are some examples of starter, eating, and exercise affirmations with photos you can choose.

I forgive myself and others for mistreating my body in the past.

I am worthy and fully capable of creating a light, healthy body.

AFFIRM & BURN!

I give myself permission to have a light, healthy body.

I believe in my ability to create a light, healthy body.

AFFIRM & BURN!

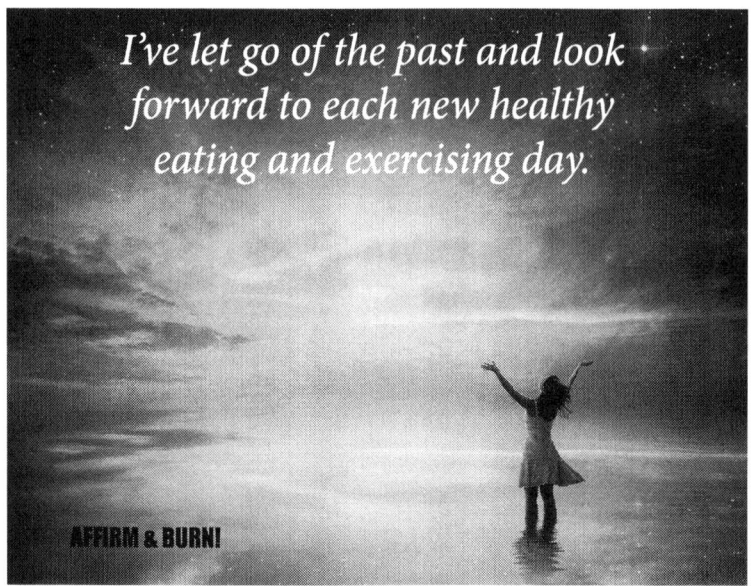

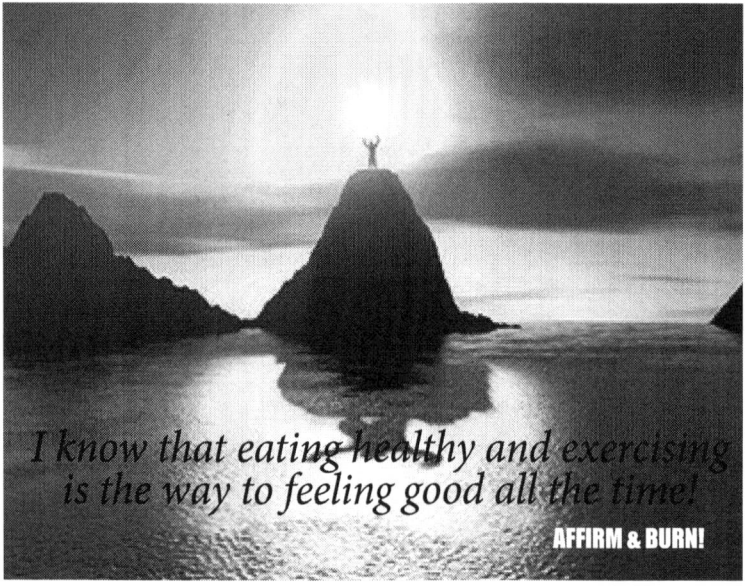

If you have more time in your schedule you may post a few of the same or different affirmations in the kitchen (on the refrigerator or cabinets) in your car, at work, etc.; anywhere you can see and read them often. Remember, the power of these affirmations increases with repetition. The more you see, read, and repeat your affirmations, out loud or in your mind, the more you will benefit. You can not do too much of this (unless the people around you begin to complain. If they do complain tell them you are simply creating a "healthy living ad campaign on yourself" the same way fast food companies do when they promote their new fattening foods). In other words, if you want to get a little crazy and fill your walls with all the affirmations like a crazed fan, go right ahead! Being a little crazy about getting yourself healthy in the beginning is good!

Some affirmations sink into the subconscious mind quickly and help you to act the way you want in a short time. That's great. Pay attention to how you are thinking and feeling to see when you feel like focusing on a different affirmation. You may decide that just one affirmation seems appropriate for a few days or a week. That is fine. Always remember the main goal is using the affirmation(s) that are truly generating a feeling inside you and getting you to consistently eat healthy and exercise.

Once again, **action** is key! Only you can understand when an affirmation has truly sunk in, causing you to act the way you want. When this happens, feel free to move on to another affirmation to address another issue you might have.

For example: If exercise has become enjoyable for you, but you find yourself struggling with food, focus more on eating affirmations.

*It is also very important to refrain from saying or thinking negatively in any way. Do not find yourself saying how much you wish you could still eat a certain fattening food or how much you still love a particular fattening food or how you do not like exercise. Don't do this even in a joking way! If you make these statements to others or agree with those who talk like this, it will only work against you. Remember that your subconscious is always listening and it does not have a sense of humor. Be aware of what you say and always choose to remain incredibly positive about eating healthy foods and exercising!

4. As soon as possible purchase a portable music device, iPod, or smartphone, etc., and create a playlist of songs that make you want to move. The playlist should be at least 30 minutes long, with the first few songs being inspirational and the latter songs being much more powerful, to get you through the tougher part of your workout. If you do not have any idea how to do this, find a teenager and pay them to do it for you. It's worth the investment! Music can be an extremely beneficial tool in getting you to move!

QUICK SUMMARY OF WHAT TO DO

Read all the affirmations, highlighting what you like most. Pick two starter affirmations, one eating affirmation, and one exercise affirmation. Memorize these (or type or say them into a cell phone if you have one) and have fun repeating them throughout the day, as often as you can. Post them on your bathroom and bedroom walls, where you work, or any where you can see and read them often. Pay attention to how you feel about eating healthier and exercising, and begin doing it daily only when you truly feel like you want to. Remember that *Affirm & Burn!* is about pleasure and choosing to eat healthy and exercise **because it makes you feel good,** not because you "think you should but don't really want to."

Create your inspiring music playlists so you will have them ready when you begin to exercise on a regular basis. The music you choose that is right for you will most definitely work as an incredible source of energy and motivation during your workouts. It will help you feel even better during your workouts.

"START OFF" AFFIRMATIONS

The affirmations below are what we will call "start off" affirmations to be used at the start (first two weeks) of your journey. They focus on your being fully committed to your health goal, compassionate with yourself, forgiving of yourself, and more mindful of the present. They will also help you to develop a higher level of self worth—a vital part of your program. Do you really feel like you deserve to be light and healthy? Are you willing to forgive yourself and others for mistakes in the past? Repeating these affirmations will help you with issues like these. Be sure to highlight or check the ones that really "click" with you.

I FORGIVE MYSELF AND OTHERS FOR MISTREATING MY BODY IN THE PAST

I KNOW I CAN SUCCEED NO MATTER WHAT HAS HAPPENED TO ME IN THE PAST

THE MISTAKES OF THE PAST ARE AN ILLUSION; MY ONLY REALITY IS NOW

I'VE LET GO OF THE PAST AND LOOK FORWARD TO EACH NEW HEALTHY EATING AND EXERCISING DAY

I GIVE MYSELF PERMISSION TO HAVE A BEAUTIFUL, HEALTHY BODY

I EXPECT FANTASTIC RESULTS AND I GET THEM

I TRUST MY ALWAYS-INCREASING ABILITY TO
CREATE A LIGHT, HEALTHY BODY

I TRUST MY ALWAYS-INCREASING ABILITY
TO BE STRONG AND FOCUSED ON MY
HEALTH AND WELL-BEING

I ACCEPT AND LOVE MY BODY RIGHT NOW

I BELIEVE IN MY ABILITY TO CREATE
A LEAN, HEALTHY BODY

I AM WILLING TO DO WHATEVER IT TAKES
TO REACH MY HEALTH GOAL

I AM TOTALLY COMMITTED TO MY GOAL
OF A LEAN, HEALTHY BODY

I AM WORTHY AND FULLY CAPABLE OF
CREATING A LEAN, HEALTHY BODY

I LOVE AND RESPECT MY BODY

MY BODY IS MIRACULOUS AND SERVES ME WELL

MY BODY IS EVER READY TO WORK WITH
ME IN BECOMING HEALTHIER

I NOW DESERVE A HEALTHY BODY

I AM EXCITED ABOUT MY BODY BECOMING LIGHTER

I BELIEVE IN MY ALWAYS-INCREASING ABILITY
TO CREATE TOTAL HEALTH

MY BODY IS MY BEST AND MOST LOYAL FRIEND

I TREAT MY BODY EXTREMELY WELL

MY BODY IS MY MOST PRIZED POSSESSION

I NOW TAKE CARE OF MY BODY
AND IT TAKES CARE OF ME

I GIVE MYSELF PERMISSION TO ENJOY
A HEALTHY LIFESTYLE

I CHOOSE TO LIVE A HEALTHY LIFE RIGHT NOW

I AM EXCITED ABOUT BECOMING LIGHTER
AND HEALTHIER EACH DAY

I KNOW I HAVE AN UNLIMITED AMOUNT
OF POWER WITHIN ME

I AM BECOMING LIGHTER AND FEELING
GREAT RIGHT NOW

I AM GETTING SLENDER AND
HEALTHIER EACH DAY

I CAN BE HEALTHIER AND HAPPIER
THAN I COULD EVER IMAGINE

I HAVE MORE WILLPOWER IN ME THAN
I COULD POSSIBLY IMAGINE

I PICTURE A LEAN, HEALTHY BODY FOR MYSELF

I DESERVE A HEALTHY BODY

MY THOUGHTS ARE FOCUSED ON THE
HEALTH OF MY BODY

I ONLY GET ONE BODY IN THIS LIFE SO
I KNOW TO TREAT IT WELL

I'M FINDING MORE AND MORE REASONS TO STAY
FOCUSED ON MY HEALTH GOALS

I KNOW THAT TAKING CARE OF MY BODY
IS ALWAYS THE RIGHT THING TO DO

I AM THRILLED BY MY NEW HEALTHY
WAY OF LIVING MY LIFE

I KNOW THAT EATING HEALTHY AND EXERCISING IS
THE WAY TO FEELING GOOD ALL THE TIME

I FEEL GOOD ABOUT ALL THE EXERCISE
I CHOOSE TO DO REGULARLY

I LOVE AND APPRECIATE MY BODY THAT HAS
BEEN WORKING FOR ME SINCE BIRTH

MY BODY IS A MIRACULOUS WORK
OF NATURE. I TREAT IT WELL

I KNOW I CAN HAVE A LIGHTER, HEALTHIER BODY

I AM EXCITED ABOUT MAKING MY BODY
AS HEALTHY AS IT CAN BE

"ALTERNATE PLEASURE" AFFIRMATIONS

Many people who are overweight or obese often got that way simply because they chose to believe, and consistently affirm consciously or unconsciously, that most of the pleasure in life comes from tasting and consuming food. It is the "live to eat" philosophy. Others might overeat or eat unnecessary foods due to boredom, loneliness, frustration, joy, or any other emotion. If this is the case for you and you want to lose weight, simply choose to begin to think of other ways of making yourself feel good.

Yes, there are actual ways to make yourself feel really good that do not always involve eating! Diversify your pleasure! Go for a walk while you talk with a friend on the phone. Don't have any friends available? Listen to an inspirational audiobook with a portable device while walking. Take a bath. Get a massage. Relax on a couch and listen to music that relaxes you as you visualize yourself looking lighter and healthier. Do some research. Talk to other people and find out what brings them pleasure besides eating.

A woman I'll call Amy learned how to do this. Here's her story:

Every time Amy (who loved to eat fast food for pleasure) drove her car and was not thinking of anything in particular she would undoubtedly see a fast food establishment. As soon as she saw the colorful building and the familiar logo, pleasant thoughts of eating the food would enter her mind, even though she was not truly hungry. Automatically, she would pull over, head for the drive thru, and be eating that food in the parking lot within minutes. After playing with affirmations for a few days, the next time she drove past a fast food restaurant she became AWARE of what was about to happen. She smiled to herself as she drove by and affirmed, "I'm happy eating only healthy food when I'm truly hungry." This simple statement rang true and seemed to keep her from pulling over. She then thought of another affirmation: "The proper eating I do is even better for me than I can possibly imagine." Soon she was home and anxious to go for a power walk and prepare a healthy meal for dinner later, when she would truly be hungry.

Remember: the following affirmations will help affirm alternatives to feeling good that do not involve unnecessary eating. Pick your favorites and repeat them during times you may be tempted to eat unnecessarily. Feel free to substitute an activity that particularly interests you, even if it's not on this list.

**I MAKE MYSELF FEEL GOOD BY TAKING A WALK
AND LISTENING TO BEAUTIFUL MUSIC**

**I CAN MAKE MYSELF FEEL GOOD
BY GETTING A MASSAGE**

**I CAN COMFORT MYSELF WITH A
MANICURE OR PEDICURE**

**I ENJOY TAKING A SOOTHING HOT BATH OR
SHOWER AT NIGHT IF I'M BORED, LONELY, OR UPSET**

**I COMFORT MYSELF BY TAKING
A WARM OR COOL BATH OR SHOWER**

**I ENJOY SIMPLY TALKING WITH SUPPORTIVE FAMILY
AND FRIENDS IF I'M BORED, LONELY, OR UPSET**

**I PAMPER AND COMFORT MYSELF BY
SPENDING TIME WITH ANIMALS**

**I MAKE MYSELF FEEL GOOD BY READING INSPIRING
BOOKS IF I'M BORED, LONELY, OR UPSET**

I MAKE MYSELF FEEL GOOD BY LISTENING
TO BEAUTIFUL MUSIC

I MAKE MYSELF FEEL GOOD BY WATCHING
INSPIRING FILMS OR VIDEOS

I MAKE MYSELF FEEL GOOD BY TAKING A
WALK IN NATURE

I STAY LIGHT AND FEEL GOOD BY STRETCHING OR
EXERCISING IF I AM BORED, LONELY, OR UPSET

I ENJOY SPENDING TIME IN NATURE

I CAN MAKE MYSELF FEEL GOOD BY DRINKING
HERBAL TEA IF I'M BORED, LONELY, OR UPSET

I CAN MAKE MYSELF FEEL GOOD AND
LIGHT BY DRINKING COOL WATER WITH LEMON
IF I'M BORED, LONELY, OR UPSET

I CAN MAKE MYSELF FEEL GOOD BY
HELPING OTHERS IN NEED

I ENJOY CREATIVE ACTIVITIES LIKE DRAWING,
PAINTING, OR SCULPTING IF I'M BORED,
LONELY, OR UPSET

I ENJOY CLEANING UP MY HOME IF I'M BORED,
LONELY, OR UPSET

I ENJOY RELEASING TENSION BY STRETCHING
MY LEG MUSCLES

I ENJOY RELEASING TENSION BY DOING YOGA

I CHEW GUM TO FEEL GOOD IF I'M FORCED TO BE
AROUND FOOD THAT COULD TEMPT ME

I LOVE USING GUM AS A WAY TO AVOID UNNECESSARY EATING

IF TEMPTING FOOD IS LEFT ON A TABLE I MUST SIT AT, I CHEW DELICIOUS GUM

"WHEN YOU SEE RESULTS AFTER A WEEK OR TWO AFFIRMATIONS"

These affirmations are for when you have dropped a few pounds and are really beginning to enjoy the process of eating healthy and exercising. They basically reaffirm why you are continuing to do what you have set out to do.

The truth is, as you choose to consistently eat foods that contain less fat or less sugar your body will adjust and start to like it! In other words, you will no longer want to eat ice cream that is not low-fat because it will taste "too fatty" for you. It will be the same with high fructose syrup drinks or foods fried in a lot of bad oil. You will find the drinks too sweet and the fried foods greasy and disgusting.

It might take a few days, or weeks but it will happen in time if you affirm and keep doing it. Trust me and give the healthy foods a chance! If they are not very tasty to you at first, eat them anyway. Keep doing it!

Every person who started a habit, such as smoking or drinking, at first probably thought it was disgusting, but they kept doing it. Think of how much easier it will be for you to eat foods that truly nourish your body if you keep eating them and affirming. When you do this you'll find the unwanted fat will drop off your body easily and effortlessly.

One last thing: you might get compliments from friends as you lose weight. That is a good source of motivation, but do not rely on that—those compliments will stop at some point. Ultimately, you must be your own source of motivation! Good health through eating healthy and exercising is all about you and what you do, not anyone else. That is how these affirmations will help you.

Switch to these affirmations or simply add them on when it feels right for you.

**I SLEEP WELL AT NIGHT KNOWING I HAD
A GREAT, HEALTHY DAY**

**I SLEEP BETTER AT NIGHT WHEN I'VE
EXERCISED DURING THE DAY**

**I LOVE BECOMING LIGHTER AND HEALTHIER
EVERY MINUTE OF THE DAY**

**I LOVE BEING LIGHTER AND ABLE TO SHOP
AT ANY STORE FOR CLOTHING**

**I TREAT MY BODY AS I WOULD A
LOVABLE, TREASURED PET**

**I LOVE FEELING MORE CONFIDENT AND HAPPY ALL
DAY LONG IN MY LIGHTER, HEALTHIER BODY**

**I LOVE HAVING MORE CONFIDENCE AND
MORE ENERGY EVERY DAY**

**I TRUST MY BODY IS DOING THE BEST IT
CAN FOR ME ALL THE TIME**

**I LOVE FEELING GOOD ABOUT THE GOOD
THINGS I'M DOING FOR MY BODY**

I LOVE THAT I'M GETTING LIGHTER, STRONGER, AND BETTER EVERY DAY

I FEEL LIGHTER, AND FEELING LIGHTER FEELS FANTASTIC

I AM MOVING TOWARD INCREASED LIGHTNESS AND ENERGY EVERY DAY

I'M GAINING MORE AND MORE LIGHTNESS AND ENERGY EVERY DAY

I'M GETTING BETTER EVERY DAY AND I'M GOING TO STAY THAT WAY

I LOVE EATING LOW-FAT FOODS AND FEELING GREAT

I CHOOSE TO EAT HEALTHIER FOOD BECAUSE IT MAKES ME FEEL BETTER

EATING HEALTHY IS SO EASY BECAUSE IT MAKES MY BODY FEEL GREAT

EATING HEALTHY AND FEELING GREAT IS MY NEW WAY OF LIFE

I CONGRATULATE MYSELF ALL DAY LONG AS I FOLLOW THE BEAUTIFUL PATH TO A LIGHTER, HEALTHIER BODY

I LOVE WAKING UP IN THE MORNING FEELING LIGHTER

I LOVE WAKING UP IN THE MORNING KNOWING I DID GREAT THE DAY BEFORE

I LOVE WAKING UP IN THE MORNING READY TO EAT PROPERLY FOR THE DAY

I KNOW THAT DEEP DOWN I HAVE ACCESS TO SUPERHUMAN STRENGTH AND ENDURANCE

I'M FINDING MORE AND MORE REASONS TO CONTINUE EATING HEALTHY AND EXERCISING EVERY DAY

I'M EATING HEALTHY, EXERCISING, AND FEELING PHENOMENAL EVERY DAY

I EAT HEALTHY AND EXERCISE BECAUSE IT MAKES ME FEEL GOOD ALL DAY LONG

"EATING AFFIRMATIONS"

These affirmations focus on eating healthy food, in proper portions, when you are truly hungry. The essence of the *Affirm & Burn!* philosophy is to constantly remind yourself that what you really want in life is to **feel good** as much as you can and that eating healthy and exercising on a regular basis is the key to consistently feeling good. Do the math! Do you want to feel good eating junk for an hour or two a day or feel great 24 hours a day leading a healthy lifestyle? (I say 24 hours because you will even sleep better when you are leaner and healthier!)

When you use the techniques in *Affirm & Burn!* and ultimately make the simple realization in your mind that eating healthy food, thinking right, and exercising regularly is the key to feeling good all the time, you simply won't go back to the temporary, shallow, joy of junk food and laziness. It will be as if you've become a "health food and exercise addict." Your body will literally learn to crave exercise and healthier foods like fruits and vegetables with a true desire to go out of your way to get them if necessary!

Eating healthy and exercising on a regular basis is a FLAWLESS, FEEL GOOD FORMULA and NATURAL HIGH that is truly what you will want to experience as often as possible. When that belief is consistently reaffirmed in your mind, the temptation to overeat or eat a fattening unhealthy snack to make yourself feel good will fade, and in time, become almost non-existent.

Use the following clever affirmations to keep that type of extremely powerful thinking in your head.

**I EAT ONLY HEALTHY FOOD
WHEN I AM TRULY HUNGRY**

**I'M HAPPY EATING ONLY HEALTHY FOOD
WHEN MY BODY IS TRULY HUNGRY**

**I LOVE EATING ONLY HEALTHY FOOD WHEN
MY BODY IS TRULY HUNGRY**

**I PLAN AND PREPARE MY HEALTHY MEALS FOR THE
WEEK AND EAT ONLY THEM.
LIFE IS SIMPLY FANTASTIC THAT WAY**

**I EAT ONLY MY PREPARED MEALS AND SNACKS
EVERY DAY AND ENJOY AS MUCH WATER AND
SUGARLESS GUM CHEWING AS I WANT**

**LIFE IS FANTASTIC, JOYOUS, AND BEAUTIFUL
WHEN I EAT ONLY MY PERFECTLY PLANNED
HEALTHY MEALS**

**I EAT ONLY HEALTHY FOOD WHEN MY BODY
TRULY NEEDS NOURISHMENT**

I EAT TO LIVE HAPPILY IN MY LEAN,
HEALTHY, MIRACULOUS, BODY

I FEEL GOOD ABOUT ALL THE HEALTHY
FOOD I CHOOSE TO EAT

MY LIFE IS ABOUT FEELING GOOD, AND EATING
HEALTHY AND EXERCISING IS THE WAY

MY BODY REALLY LOVES EATING HEALTHY FOOD

EATING HEALTHY FOOD IN PROPER PORTIONS
MAKES ME FEEL AMAZING, AND I AM AMAZING

EATING HEALTHY PROPER PORTIONS MEANS
MORE ENERGY AND HAPPINESS FOR ME

I KNOW EATING SIMPLE, HEALTHY, MEALS ALWAYS
MAKES ME FEEL FANTASTIC IN EVERY WAY

I LOVE EATING SIMPLE, HEALTHY, MEALS IN
PROPER PORTIONS EVERY DAY

I ENJOY EATING WHEN I AM TRULY HUNGRY, CALM,
AND AT EASE WITH MYSELF

I CARE MORE ABOUT THE HEALTH OF THE
FOOD THAN THE TASTE

I AM IN COMPLETE CONTROL OF
EVERYTHING I EAT

EATING HEALTHIER MAKES GOING TO THE
BATHROOM EASIER

I ENJOY THE HEALTHFULNESS OF THE FOOD MUCH
MORE THAN THE TASTE

I KNOW THAT I WANT TO FEEL GOOD MOST OF
THE TIME, AND EATING RIGHT AND EXERCISING
IS THE KEY

I CONGRATULATE MYSELF OFTEN FOR
MAKING GREAT FOOD CHOICES

SMALL HEALTHY MEALS MEANS MORE TIME,
MONEY, AND ENERGY FOR ME

I LOVE AND APPRECIATE THE EXTRA TIME
AND MONEY I SAVE BY EATING LESS.
LESS REALLY IS MORE!

MY BODY FEELS FANTASTIC WHEN I EAT
HEALTHY MEALS EVERY DAY

I ALWAYS LOOK FOR WAYS TO HELP OTHERS TO
EAT HEALTHIER; AS I HELP THEM, I HELP MYSELF

I MAKE PROPER FOOD CHOICES BECAUSE
I LOVE MY BODY AND MY LIFE

MY HOME IS FILLED ONLY WITH HEALTHY FOODS
AND I LOVE IT THAT WAY

I KNOW THAT EATING HEALTHY FOOD
MAKES ME FEEL GOOD ALL THE TIME

I TREAT MY BODY LIKE AN EXPENSIVE AUTOMOBILE,
GIVING IT ONLY THE PERFECT AMOUNT OF QUALITY
FOOD FUEL EVERY DAY

FRUITS, VEGETABLES, PROTEIN, AND
WHOLE GRAINS KEEP ME FEELING FANTASTIC
24 HOURS A DAY

MY BODY IS A PART OF NATURE. I ENJOY EATING
MORE NATURAL FOODS AS MUCH AS I CAN

I CHOOSE TO EAT SMALL PORTIONS OF FRESH
FRUIT, HEALTHY NUTS, OR SEEDS AS SNACKS

I CHOOSE TO EAT SMALL PORTIONS OF WHOLE
GRAIN CRACKERS OR FRUITS AS SNACKS

I LOVE SATISFYING HUNGER PAINS WITH HIGH
PROTEIN, LOW-FAT, AND FIBROUS FOOD

I LOVE A SMOOTH, SMALL, CREAMY, LOW-FAT
YOGURT AS A SNACK

I CONSTANTLY REMEMBER HOW GOOD MY BODY
FEELS ALL DAY LONG FROM EATING PROPER
PORTIONS OF HEALTHY, NATURAL, FOOD

I AM BECOMING A HEALTH FOOD ADDICT AND
LOVING EVERY MINUTE OF IT

MY HOME HAS ONLY HEALTHY, NATURAL FOODS IN
IT BECAUSE MY BODY IS HEALTHY AND NATURAL

I CONGRATULATE MYSELF OFTEN FOR MAKING
EXCELLENT HEALTHY FOOD CHOICES

I FEEL SO POWERFUL WHEN I MAKE
PROPER FOOD CHOICES

I LOVE TO EAT HEALTHY FOOD THAT
MAKES MY BODY FEEL GOOD

I ALWAYS LEAVE SOME FOOD ON MY PLATE. BIRDS
AND BUGS AT THE LANDFILL MUST EAT TOO

I LOVE THAT I NOW CHOOSE TO WALK AWAY
FROM MY MAIN MEALS 3/4 FULL

I PAY FULL ATTENTION TO EVERYTHING
THAT GOES INTO MY MOUTH

I FULLY UNDERSTAND THAT I ALONE AM
ALWAYS 100% RESPONSIBLE FOR WHAT AND
HOW MUCH I EAT

100% RESPONSIBILITY MEANS I HAVE
ALL THE POWER AND I LOVE THAT

IF I MUST CHEAT, I CHEAT AS SMALL AS POSSIBLE
AND TAKE FULL RESPONSIBILITY FOR IT

IF I OVEREAT ONE DAY I KNOW I ENJOY EATING
LESS AND EXERCISING MORE THE VERY NEXT DAY

I REMEMBER HOW TERRIBLE I FEEL
PHYSICALLY IF I MISTAKENLY OVEREAT

IF I MISTAKENLY OVEREAT, I KNOW I WON'T
DO IT AGAIN FOR A LONG TIME

IF I MISTAKENLY OVEREAT, MY NEXT TWO
MEALS WILL BE EXTRA SMALL

MY NEW INCREDIBLE HEALTHY EATING HABITS ARE
SETTING AN AWESOME EXAMPLE FOR OTHERS

I OBEY THE HIGHER, WISER, PART OF MY MIND
WHEN MAKING FOOD CHOICES

WHEN I'M EATING OUT WITH FRIENDS I
CHOOSE TO EAT SLOWLY, PROPERLY, AND
WITH FULL ATTENTION

I LOVE ALWAYS BEING FULLY AWARE AND IN
CONTROL OF WHAT I AM EATING

I ALWAYS ENJOY MY MEALS MORE WHEN I EAT
WITH FULL ATTENTION

I'M ALWAYS FULLY AWARE OF EVERYTHING
I PUT IN MY MOUTH

I LOVE GOING FOR LONG, RELAXING,
WALKS AFTER MY MEALS

I SKIP FATTENING DESSERTS, PREFERRING A
PLEASANT CONVERSATION, A WALK, OR BOTH

THE NEW ME IS HEALTHY

THE PROPER EATING I DO IS EVEN BETTER
FOR ME THAN I CAN POSSIBLY IMAGINE

MY HEALTHY EATING AND EXERCISE
HABITS ELECTRIFY MY SPIRIT

MY NEW HEALTHY LIFESTYLE IS THE REAL
HAPPINESS I'VE BEEN SEEKING

I ALWAYS CHOOSE TO EAT HEALTHY FOODS
THAT TRULY NOURISH MY BODY

I LOVE EATING FRUITS AND VEGETABLES

I KNOW THAT THE FEEL GOOD LIFE FORCE
COMES FROM FRUITS, VEGETABLES, WHOLE
GRAINS, AND OTHER HEALTHY FOODS

WHEN I'M EATING OUT WITH FRIENDS I ENJOY
THE ATMOSPHERE AND THEIR COMPANY AND
WILL NOT EAT UNLESS I AM TRULY HUNGRY

**AFTER DINNER I ENJOY CHEWING TASTY
GUM OVER DESSERT**

**I'M EATING HEALTHY, EXERCISING,
AND FEELING MORE FANTASTIC EVERY DAY**

**I'M EXPERIENCING INCREDIBLE LIGHTNESS,
HEALTH, AND ENERGY EATING ONLY
MY PERFECTLY PLANNED MEALS**

**MY BODY IS LIKE A PERFECT MACHINE
EATING HEALTHY MEALS, EXERCISING,
AND FEELING FANTASTIC**

**I CONGRATULATE MYSELF OFTEN FOR
MAKING GREAT FOOD CHOICES**

"AFFIRMATIONS FOR TROUBLING SITUATIONS"

These affirmations will help those of you who may be forced into social situations that could sabotage your success. You may have friends, coworkers, clients, or family members who are not interested or do not need to get light and healthy. They might ridicule you, call you a "health nut," tell you to "relax and enjoy life," etc. That's fine. Don't get angry or frustrated. Remain calm, smile, and send them love. This is the best way to deal with the situation. If you can do this and keep your sense of humor, you will be fine. In time, you will most likely find the same people soon wanting to follow your amazing example of how to live a healthy lifestyle!

Some of the affirmations listed here can also help as playful responses to those who may try to sabotage you. Keeping your sense of humor in troubling or tempting situations can be most powerful.

I CHEW GUM IF I'M FORCED TO BE AROUND BAD
FOOD OR PEOPLE WHO COULD TEMPT ME

I LOVE USING GUM AS A WAY TO AVOID
UNNECESSARY EATING

IF TEMPTING FOOD IS LEFT ON A TABLE I MUST
SIT AT, I CHEW DELICIOUS GUM

I ALWAYS KEEP A PACK OF SUGARLESS
GUM WITH ME

I USE GUM AS A POWERFUL TOOL TO
AVOID UNNECESSARY EATING

IT'S MY MOUTH AND MY STOMACH. NO ONE CAN
FORCE ME TO PUT EXTRA OR UNHEALTHY FOOD
IN IT WITHOUT MY PERMISSION

I POLITELY EXCUSE MYSELF FROM OTHERS
WHO MAY WANT TO SABOTAGE MY PATH
TO LIGHTNESS AND GREAT HEALTH

I REMAIN CALM AND STRONG WITHIN
IF OTHERS TRY TO TEMPT ME

IF, ON OCCASION, NOTHING BUT UNHEALTHY
FATTENING FOOD IS AVAILABLE, I WILL
EAT AS LITTLE OF IT AS POSSIBLE

MY WILL IS SO STRONG AND I FEEL SO GOOD THAT
NO ONE CAN MAKE ME EAT IMPROPERLY

I SMILE CALMLY AND CONFIDENTLY AND SEND LOVE
TO THOSE WHO MAY WANT ME TO EAT THE WRONG
FOOD OR TOO MUCH FOOD

I EAT HEALTHY FOOD IN PROPER PORTIONS
EVEN WHEN I OR FRIENDS REALLY FEEL
LIKE PIGGING OUT

I EAT HEALTHY FOOD IN PROPER PORTIONS EVEN
WHEN I AM AT A PARTY OR CELEBRATION

I EAT HEALTHY FOOD IN PROPER PORTIONS
EVEN WHEN I REALLY FEEL LIKE CHEATING

I NOW CHOOSE TO WASTE EXTRA,
UNNECESSARY FOOD IN THE GARBAGE CAN,
THAN TO WASTE IT ON ME

I NOW BELIEVE IT IS WRONG TO FORCE MYSELF
TO EAT EXTRA FOOD JUST BECAUSE IT WILL BE
THROWN AWAY OR OTHERS WANT ME TO

Here are some silly but powerful rhyme responses you can have fun using on those who may try to sabotage you.

Don't you tempt me, I'm doing great, I don't need junk food, or extra weight!

I am focused and I am strong, leaner and lighter, all day long!

Leaner and lighter, feeling great, healthier and happier, that's my fate!

I just do, what needs to be done, I look great, and I have fun!

I just do, what needs to be done, I feel great, and I have fun!

Sticking to the program, I have the power, getting lighter, every hour!

Eating right, is no big deal, after all, it's just a meal!

There's more to life, than tons of food, other things, can lift my mood!

Good health is key, there's no debate, the goal is perfect, and it feels great!

I love to eat, healthy meals, because I like, the way it feels!

EXERCISE AFFIRMATIONS

These affirmations will help you to exercise more. If you struggle with eating and truly find it absolutely impossible to eat proper portions or to avoid certain fattening foods most of the time then you must exercise more to make up for it!

Exercise CAN BE ENJOYABLE! There are so many good things that happen to your mind and body when you exercise regularly. According to the latest research, exercising regularly gives you more energy, makes you look better, sleep better, releases stress, helps your immune system, and overall makes you a happier person. Many people do indeed get addicted to exercise once they realize that all of that is true. The affirmations that follow will help you realize that.

Please note that there are a few affirmations here that seem to go against the basic philosophy of this program. In the introduction of this book, I explained how powerful your mind is when it comes to doing anything. This is true, but when it comes to acting on something, particularly exercise, the body can lead the mind and act without its permission. In other words, the mind can suddenly change and be led by the body first, once the body is in motion. Sir Isaac Newton, the brilliant English physicist, said, "An object in motion tends to stay in motion." You could also say, in terms of getting yourself to exercise, that "a human body in motion tends to stay in motion" too!

For example, you are sitting in a chair at a party with no intention of getting up. Someone physically drags you by the arm and forces you to dance and suddenly your mind changes as a result of your physical movements. You start to enjoy dancing! This is a case of the body leading the mind.

Another example is smiling! Try this as a test. Stand up straight with your shoulders back and put a big smile on your face. Then, without changing your posture or your smile, think depressing thoughts. It will be hard—almost impossible—to actually feel depressed if you do not change your posture and get rid of your smile! This is an example of how the body can lead the mind. To make these affirmations have even more power, (especially when you are feeling lazy or depressed), put your body in the most confident position you can think of, standing up straight with your shoulders back, like a superhero, and confidently say the following affirmations.

**I LOVE TO EXERCISE BECAUSE IT
MAKES ME FEEL GOOD**

I OFTEN BEGIN EXERCISING WITHOUT A REASON

**I EXERCISE EVEN WHEN I REALLY
FEEL LIKE BEING LAZY**

**MY BODY CAN ALWAYS BEGIN EXERCISING
EVEN WHEN I REALLY FEEL LIKE BEING LAZY**

**MY BODY CAN ALWAYS BEGIN EXERCISING
WITHOUT PERMISSION FROM MY MIND'S LAZY
THOUGHTS**

**I NOW EXERCISE WHEN I AM BORED,
LONELY, OR UPSET**

I'M FINDING MORE AND MORE JOY IN WORKING OUT

**I'M FINDING MORE AND MORE
REASONS TO STAY ACTIVE**

**I'M FINDING CREATIVE WAYS TO
EXERCISE WITH MY KIDS**

**I'M FINDING CREATIVE WAYS TO
BRISKLY WALK MORE TO AND FROM WORK**

I ENJOY WALKING A FEW MINUTES MORE
TO AND FROM LUNCH

I LOVE THE WAY I FEEL DURING AND
AFTER EXERCISE

I LOVE TAKING A WALK AFTER MEALS

EXERCISING IS AS EASY AND NORMAL
AS GOING TO THE BATHROOM

EXERCISING IS AS EASY AND NORMAL
AS BRUSHING MY TEETH

EXERCISING ON A REGULAR BASIS KEEPS ME
IN TUNE WITH THE INFINITE FEEL-GOOD
LIFE FORCE OF THE COSMOS

I BRING LOVE AND A POSITIVE ATTITUDE
TO ALL MY WORKOUTS

I CAN ALWAYS MAKE EXERCISING FUN IF
I CHOOSE TO

MY WORKOUTS BEGIN EASILY WITH
FANTASTIC, POSITIVE THOUGHTS

I THINK OF EMPOWERING, ENERGIZING, THOUGHTS
TO GET ME EXCITED ABOUT EXERCISE

I THINK OF EMPOWERING, ENERGIZING, THOUGHTS
THROUGHOUT MY WORKOUTS

GREAT, EMPOWERING, POSITIVE THOUGHTS CAN
ALWAYS GIVE ME ENERGY

I LOVE THE WAY MY MIND BECOMES CRYSTAL
CLEAR AND FOCUSED DURING THE MOST
INTENSE PART OF MY WORKOUTS

I CONGRATULATE MYSELF AFTER EVERY WORKOUT

I ALWAYS REMEMBER HOW GREAT I
FEEL AFTER ANY WORKOUT

EXERCISING REGULARLY IS THE
SECRET TO HAPPINESS

EXERCISING REGULARLY IS THE
SECRET TO BETTER SLEEP

HAPPINESS COMES FROM EATING
HEALTHY AND EXERCISING

I MOTIVATE MYSELF TO EXERCISE BY USING
POWERFUL, POSITIVE THOUGHTS

I MOTIVATE MYSELF TO EXERCISE BY USING
ELECTRIFYING, EXHILARATING MUSIC

EXERCISING UPLIFTS MY MOOD AND MAKES ME
FEEL FANTASTIC BOTH PHYSICALLY AND MENTALLY

EXERCISING WITH ENERGIZING MUSIC
INVIGORATES MY MIND AND BODY

I KNOW THE KIND OF EXERCISE
I LOVE TO DO AND I DO IT

I ALWAYS FIND SIMPLE WAYS THROUGHOUT
THE DAY TO MOVE MORE

I LOVE CHOOSING STAIRS OVER
ELEVATORS AND ESCALATORS

CLIMBING STAIRS IS FUN AND MAKES ME
FEEL YOUNG

I ENJOY PARKING MY CAR FAR FROM MY
DESTINATION SO I CAN WALK MORE

EXERCISING HELPS ME SLEEP LIKE A BABY
AT NIGHT

I LOOK FORWARD TO EATING HEALTHY,
EXERCISING, AND FEELING BETTER EVERY DAY

MY BODY LOVES AND APPRECIATES
THE EXERCISE I GIVE IT

MY BODY REWARDS ME WITH A
WONDERFULLY RELAXING FEELING AFTER
EACH INTENSE WORKOUT

I LOVE THE FEELING OF ACCOMPLISHMENT
AFTER A GOOD AEROBIC WORKOUT

I ALWAYS REMEMBER HOW GREAT IT IS TO
FEEL TIRED, CALM, AND RELAXED AFTER AN
INTENSE WORKOUT

I ALWAYS REMEMBER HOW GREAT EXERCISE
IS FOR RELEASING STRESS

THE TOUGHER THE WORKOUT, THE MORE PROUD
AND RELAXED I WILL FEEL AFTERWARDS

I REWARD MYSELF WITH A BEAUTIFUL SHOWER
OR BATH AFTER A TOUGH WORKOUT

I REMEMBER TO SMILE CONFIDENTLY AT THE
TOUGHEST POINT OF MY WORKOUT

EATING HEALTHY AND EXERCISING EACH DAY
IS MAKING ME HIGH ALL THE TIME

NIGHTTIME AFFIRMATIONS AND "JUST BEFORE YOU SLEEP" AFFIRMATIONS

Many people have difficulty avoiding unhealthy food, fattening food, or overeating at night. Ice cream, cookies, potato chips, etc. can be very tempting if they are in your home. If they can't be removed be sure to have healthy alternatives available like low-fat yogurt, low-fat cheese, fruit, whole grain crackers, nuts, or low-fat cookies etc. The following affirmations will help.

IF I'M HUNGRY AT NIGHT I DRINK COOL, FRESH, FILLING, WATER BEFORE I EAT A SMALL HEALTHY SNACK

I USE GUM AS A POWERFUL TOOL TO AVOID UNHEALTHY SNACKING AT NIGHT

I LOVE EATING ONLY A HEALTHY SNACK AT NIGHT TO SATISFY A HUNGRY FEELING

I SIMPLY REFUSE TO EAT UNHEALTHY SNACK FOOD AT NIGHT NO MATTER WHAT

I LOVE BRUSHING MY TEETH AT NIGHT AS AN END TO MY EATING FOR THE DAY

I LOVE BRUSHING, FLOSSING, AND RINSING MY TEETH WITH MOUTHWASH AS THE PERFECT END TO PERFECT EATING FOR THE DAY

I HAVE NO DESIRE TO EAT AT NIGHT AFTER I'VE BRUSHED, FLOSSED AND RINSED

Just before you sleep:

**WHEN I EAT SMALL HEALTHY PORTIONS
I SLEEP MUCH BETTER**

**EATING HEALTHY AND EXERCISING EACH DAY IS
MAKING ME SLEEP MUCH BETTER**

**I ALLOW MYSELF TO THINK AND DREAM ABOUT
A LEANER, HEALTHIER BODY**

**I ENJOY VISUALIZING A LEAN, PERFECTLY HEALTHY
BODY AS I DRIFT OFF TO SLEEP**

**I SLEEP LIKE A BABY KNOWING I MADE GREAT
CHOICES THROUGHOUT THE DAY**

**I WAS A WINNER TODAY AND WILL BE
A WINNER TOMORROW**

**I LOVE SLEEPING BETTER, WAKING UP LIGHTER,
AND HAVING MORE ENERGY EVERY DAY**

A HEALTHY BODY IS MY BIRTHRIGHT

I CHOOSE TO LIVE A HEALTHY LIFESTYLE

SPIRITUAL AFFIRMATIONS

Some people naturally become more spiritual when they begin to take care of and heal their body. For those of you who are religious or spiritually oriented, below are what we will call "spiritual affirmations" or "health prayers." They do not correspond to any particular religion or belief system. We all have our individual beliefs. Feel free to substitute any word in these affirmations that you feel more comfortable with when you see the words "God" or

"Spirit," such as the "Universe," "Christ," "the Lord," etc. You may even skip these if you like. It's up to you.

MY BODY IS FILLED WITH LOVE AND LIGHT

I AM ONE WITH THE INFINITE, INEXHAUSTIBLE SPIRIT INSIDE THIS BODY

MY BODY'S ENERGY ULTIMATELY COMES FROM THE UNIVERSAL LIFE FORCE

MY BODY'S ENERGY ULTIMATELY COMES FROM THE CREATOR

I EAT HEALTHY FOOD AND EXERCISE BECAUSE MY BODY IS MY TEMPLE

MY BODY IS A VEHICLE FOR SPIRIT. I TREAT IT WELL

I AM ONE WITH THE INFINITE POWER AND KNOW I CAN ACHIEVE ANYTHING

I CONNECT WITH AND GET UNLIMITED SUPPORT FROM GOD WHENEVER I NEED IT

AEROBIC EXERCISE MAKES ME FEEL MORE CONNECTED TO MY CREATOR

I KNOW THAT ULTIMATELY I AM NOT THE BODY. I AM AN INFINITE SPIRIT; BUT WHILE I'M IN THIS BODY I WILL TAKE GOOD CARE OF IT

I CAN FEEL THE INFINITE POWER OF GOD WORKING THROUGH ME

I WORK WITH THE INFINITE, INVISIBLE, INEXHAUSTIBLE, POWER

I KNOW THAT ALL GOOD THINGS ARE POSSIBLE

**I AM ONE WITH THE UNLIMITED
POWER OF THE UNIVERSE**

**I PICTURE MYSELF FILLED WITH COLORFUL
LIGHT DURING MY WORKOUTS**

**I AM LIGHT. I FEEL LIGHTER AND STRONGER
EVERY DAY**

**I FEEL DIVINE LIGHT IN EVERY CELL IN MY
BODY AND I FEEL GREAT**

FUN, HEALTH, POWER-RHYME AFFIRMATIONS

Rhyme affirmations that sound like a song are an excellent way to affect your subconscious mind (little kid in you). Little kids love rhymes and rhymes sink easily into the subconscious. They can be even more powerful than standard affirmations.

Have you ever had a silly, meaningless song or rhyme from a commercial that you could not get out of your head? Of course you have, especially if you heard it early in the day. That's how these fun, health, power-rhymes work. Pick your favorites and let their magic work on you. Sing one in the shower every morning!

Some can also be playful responses to people who may be a bad influence on you. So have fun and use the power rhymes!

I eat right and exercise, every day, I'm feeling great, in every way!

I'm getting lighter, every day, I'm feeling great, in every way!

I'm eating healthy, I'm eating light, it feels so good, it feels so right!

I have a perfect body, in a perfect way, I eat right and exercise, every day!

I love my body, I'm feeling great, I'm dropping pounds, I'm losing weight!

I start the day, losing weight, and stay that way, just feeling great!

Getting healthy, day by day, I make it easy, my own way!

Exercise is great, every day, I make it fun, in every way!

I just eat healthy, I just eat right, there is no war, there is no fight!

I eat right and exercise, I'm in the zone, my will is solid, like a stone!

I can do it, I know I can, I'm my own, biggest fan!

Feeling great, lifting weights, getting toner, and more dates!

I'm light and lean, I've got the look, wait till they see me, on Facebook!

I'm leaner and lighter, I know I am, wait till they see me, on Instagram!

I eat right and exercise, work is play, I'm feeling great, in every way!

I love exercise, it loves me, feeling great, that's the key!

Exercise is awesome, it releases stress, and ensures, a good night's rest!

I'm burning calories, I'm getting thinner, I'm feeling great, I am a winner!

After work, I just can't wait, cause exercise feels, oh so great!

I love getting up, every day, cause I succeed, in every way!

I run, I walk, I walk, and run, I just keep moving, until I'm done!

I laugh and play, I dance and sing, I find joy in everything!

Life is beautiful, so much to learn, I'm active now, and the calories burn!

I always leave, some food on my plate, better there, than extra weight!

My tummy's flatter, my butt is small, I'm looking great, and having a ball!

If I'm tempted, I walk away, I know I'll get, through this day!

Stronger and lighter every day, it just gets easier, in every way!

I won't be tempted, I will not fall, I'm strong and powerful, I make the call!

I'm smart, I'm good, I'm strong and tough, I know I've got, the right stuff!

I keep junk, away from me, I can't eat, what I can't see!

So many drinks, so hard to pick, but not for me, water's the trick!

Strong and lean, fit and cool, wait and see me, at the pool!

I'm fit and lean, it's in my reach, wait and see me, at the beach!

I love to move, to sing and play, I look forward, to every day!

I truly love, living healthy, that's the way, to being wealthy!

Who needs junk food? No, not me. Keep that crap away from me!

I love to move, and sweat, and play, my new found life, is A O.K.!

Low-fat ice cream, low-fat cheese, these are foods that aim to please!

I can't get enough, of this healthy lifestyle, I wanna go, the extra mile!

Getting leaner, makes me smile, I now wear clothes, with lots of style!

Light is in, and that is me, feeling great, that's the key!

My will is sturdy, mighty, and strong, I have great willpower, all day long!

If I fall and overeat, I know tomorrow, I won't be beat!

If I mess up, it's OK, I'll be on track, the next day!

While you are working out:

I will reach my healthy weight, and I will stay there, looking great!

I run, I run, I'm having fun, I will not stop till I am done!

I'm moving fast and breathing hard, I know I'm dropping, lots of lard!

I keep moving, I will not stop, this extra weight, I must drop!

I truly love, healthy food, it keeps me in, a great mood!

Infinite power, inside of me, supremely happy, and filled with glee!

Unlimited energy, in my veins, I feel fantastic, there are no pains!

Healthy, healthy, I feel so right, my body is, so strong and light!

CHAPTER 4

WORKOUT JOY-POWER WORDS!

Words/phrases/statements have power and can give or take energy away from us. Many people sadly think of words that give little or no power, especially during exercise. You may have said or thought the following during your workout:

"I'm exhausted. How much longer? I can't go on. I'm so tired. This is horrible! I'll never make it.

I hate exercise! I can't do any more! It's too much!

Of course, these thoughts or keywords in the thoughts, made your workout much more difficult than it had to be! (Get a pen and cross out the words above right now. Never read or say them again!) The truth is, if certain words can take energy away from you, there must be words that can give you incredible energy. I call them power thoughts or joy-power words!

The joy-power statements are special. Use them on these special occasions:

1) Those days when you're feeling very lazy or tired and do not feel like exercising.

2) During any workout when you are "hitting the wall" and feel like you just cannot go on.

3) When you really want to increase your metabolism through more intense interval workouts.

Directions: Say (or think) four joy-power statements at a time, with feeling, when you are feeling lazy or need an extra burst of energy during a workout. Start with number 1. Repeat each line at least three times before moving to the next line. You may rearrange the words if you like. You can also read them into your phone or another recording device and play them back to yourself, or have your smartphone read them to you. Whatever feels most inspiring and energizing to you is right!

I AM:

1) ENERGIZED, EXCITED, EXHILARATED, ENTHRALLED!

2) REMARKABLE, RESILIENT, RIVETED, READY!

3) POWERFUL, IMPRESSIVE, OUTRAGEOUS, GREAT!

4) AWESOME, FABULOUS, INCREDIBLE, AMAZING!

5) STRONG, A SUPERHERO, GOD-LIKE, UNSTOPPABLE!

6) UNLIMITED, UNBEATABLE, UNBELIEVABLE, INVINCIBLE!

7) VICTORIOUS, WINNING, PERFECT, SENSATIONAL!

8) SPUNKY, DYNAMIC, SPIRITED, WONDERFUL!

9) PASSIONATE, SEXY, SEDUCTIVE, BEAUTIFUL!

10) HEALTHY, HAPPY, SMILING, BLISSFUL!

11) INFINITE, ETERNAL, EVERLASTING, INEXHAUSTIBLE!

12) AWESOME, INCREDIBLE, ASTOUNDING, AMAZING!

13) MIRACULOUS, SUPERNATURAL, STUPENDOUS, WONDROUS!

14) IMPRESSIVE, OUTSTANDING, SPECTACULAR, SENSATIONAL!

15) TERRIFIC, EXCELLENT, PERFECT, EXTRAORDINARY!

16) MARVELOUS, GLORIOUS, IRREPRESSIBLE, SUPERB!

17) INVIGORATED, STIMULATED, ENLIVENED, ENTHUSED!

18) PHENOMENAL, FANTASTIC, FORCEFUL, FORMIDABLE!

19) BRIGHTENED, MOTIVATED, DETERMINED, DRIVEN!

20) MAGNIFICENT, PROUD, SPLENDID, GLORIOUS!

WORKOUT JOY-POWER PHRASES!

Directions: Choose the phrase you like most and repeat it in your mind or out loud during your aerobic workout. Whichever phrase gives you more energy is the right one!

1)   **LOOKING GREAT,**
     FEELING GREAT,
     I AM GREAT,
     LIFE IS GREAT!

2)   **LOOKING BETTER,**
     FEELING BETTER,
     GETTING BETTER,
     LIFE IS BETTER!

3)   **I HAVE ENERGY,**
     I FEEL ENERGY,
     I AM ENERGY,
     LIFE IS ENERGY!

4)   **I HAVE THE POWER,**
     I FEEL THE POWER,
     I LOVE THE POWER,
     I AM THE POWER!

If you used the joy-power statements and phrases during your workout, you probably noticed a feeling of extra power or an uplift in your mood. You may have even wanted to exercise longer. That is what the joy-power words and phrases do. They are amazing!

They can be even more powerful if you say them while listening to music. Choose music that inspires you. Experiment!

CHAPTER 5

THE GREAT QUESTIONS LIST

The questions below are fantastic questions to ask yourself to put you in a great mood and keep yourself motivated. You can ask yourself these questions any time you like. They work very much like the affirmations. Introduce them into your routine after the first week or two when you are very familiar with all the affirmations, because most of the answers to these questions are in the affirmations.

1. Why is getting lighter and healthier so much easier now?

2. How can I make the process of getting light and healthy even easier?

3. Why does eating only healthy food keep making me feel better and better every day?

4. Why am I losing all my desire for junk food?

5. Why is it silly and pointless to eat unhealthy?

6. Why is exercise becoming more fun every day?

7. Why is exercise making me feel good?

8. How can I make exercise more fun and easier?

9. Why am I sleeping better at night?

10. Why am I feeling more confident every day?

11. Why do I like saying my affirmations with real feeling?

12. What can I do to make myself feel good that does not involve eating unnecessary food?

13. Why do I now eat to live instead of live to eat?

14. Why do I treat my body and mind so well every day?

15. Why am I feeling better now than I have ever felt before?

16. How can I eat healthy, exercise, and feel good naturally for the rest of my life?

CHAPTER 6

What to Eat and What Not to Eat

There is so much information available today regarding nutrition. It can get very confusing! Many weight loss programs like Weight Watchers, Nutrisystem, and Jenny Craig, can tell you everything you need to know regarding what to eat and what not to eat. Some programs will even provide the healthy meals for you.

There are also many books that can tell you the exact fat and calorie content of many different types of prepared food. I highly recommend you read as many books as you can on the subject (preferably those written by doctors who specialize in weight loss) or join any program you and your doctor feel comfortable with. You can also get plenty of useful information absolutely free via the Internet or library. Each of us is different so experiment, pay close attention to your body, and see what works best for you. However, if you're not interested in doing any of the above, here are several simple approaches to eating that may work for you.

Some General Rules:

1) Weight loss is mostly about eating.

Yes, you need to exercise to burn calories, but the truth is that it is a lot easier to eat fewer calories than it is to burn them off. You burn about 250 to 300 calories doing a high impact aerobic exercise for approximately 30 minutes. To lose one pound you need to burn 3,500 calories—that is twelve, 30-minute, high-impact workouts! So the next time you want to eat a very fattening snack, think of the price you must pay in exercise!

2) Avoid eating out as much as possible.

The simple logic here is that you don't always know what you're eating when you eat out, and there can be a lot more calories in your food than you would ever expect. So...

3) Plan and prepare your meals.

Pick one or two nights a week where you can relax, plan, prepare, and freeze or refrigerate your meals and snacks for at least three to five days (or more) in advance. This is very important! The less you have to think about what you will eat throughout the day, the easier it will be for you. Cook all of your chicken breasts, boil your eggs, make little plastic bags of healthy snacks (nuts, whole grain crackers, popcorn, apples, low-fat cheese, etc.) and make sure you measure everything! Purchase several measuring cups and a scale, and know what a proper serving size is.

For example: a serving size of chicken breast, lean meat, or fish is three ounces—about the size of a deck of cards. A serving size of fruit is about the size of a baseball. A serving of vegetables is about half that. Also be sure to buy as much prepared, frozen, or canned food as possible so you will always have it on those days when you are too busy to prepare your lunch or snacks. Moreover, make sure you have those diet nutrition bars, meal replacement (protein) drinks, etc. in your closet and at your workplace just in case you have no time and need to eat. Be prepared!

Remember that ultimately, it's all in your mind! Repeat your affirmations to stay strong, focused, and positive as you follow these general rules.

Several Approaches to Diet

The "No Junk Food" Diet

Some people can lose weight by simply eliminating all junk food (see the "Bad Stuff" list) particularly fattening drinks (like sodas and coffees with added cream and sugar) and replacing them with low-fat or healthier substitutes. Example: a small serving of low-fat ice cream instead of a large serving of fattening ice cream. Water instead of soda. Get it? If this applies to you, try using this simple method at first.

The "Eat Whatever You Want But Exercise Like a Nut" Diet

Some people simply love to eat anything and everything and refuse to stop but are young and exercise so much (like Olympic athletes, professional basketball players, etc.) that they are able to maintain a healthy weight. If you are older and significantly overweight, this method is unlikely to work for you. Once you get to your ideal weight, however, you may be able to experiment with this. It all comes down to keeping track of the calories you take in and the calories you burn off.

The "Eat Half of What You Normally Eat Each Day" Diet

Do this, and replace the other half with a salad or vegetables. For example, if you eat four slices of pizza for lunch, eat only two and have a salad. If you eat two cheeseburgers, eat one, and a salad. Get it?

Nutrisystem, Weight Watchers, Jenny Craig, etc.

I'm sure you've seen the advertisements. Many people succeed with these programs, so they might be right and more convenient for you if they fit into your budget. They work just fine with *Affirm*

& Burn! and I would recommend any of these programs you and your doctor choose.

Good Ol' Calorie Counting

This scientific approach to weight loss works well for some people. There are about 3,500 calories in one pound of stored body fat. That means if you eat less and/or exercise enough to reduce your calorie intake by 3,500, you will lose one pound. Usually, about three-quarters of that pound is fat, and one quarter is lean body tissue. To lose fat, try reducing your calories by a minimum of 500, but no more than 1,000 below your maintenance level. You can find out how many calories it takes to lose weight or maintain your weight by going online and entering your personal information into a calorie calculator. A calorie calculator site is an excellent way to find out how many calories you need to eat to lose or maintain your weight. The site will also tell you the calorie content of just about every food you could think of. It's an amazing resource!

Reducing your calories by a minimum of 500 is easy to do when you simply eliminate foods from the bad list and replace them with foods from the good list!

The *Affirm & Burn!* Philosophy

Say your affirmations often so you train your mind and body first to love eating healthy food in proper portions as well as exercising.

Eat only good healthy food, about four to five small healthy meals throughout the day, when you are truly hungry. Keep track of all the calories you are consuming, and if you are truly hungry at night or in between meals, always eat healthy low-calorie snacks.

Refuse to overeat and learn to love curbing your hunger with small protein snacks and getting enough fiber in your diet. Also remember to drink plenty of water and exercise at least three times (150 to 200 minutes in total) a week. That's it!

The Good Stuff

It's a good idea to give the good foods appealing names or describe them in more appealing ways. Make up some of your own if you like. It helps! That's why advertisers do it.

Fresh fantastic fruits (organic when possible).

Vegetables (organic when possible, eaten raw, steamed, or baked) like beautiful broccoli, astounding asparagus, super celery, cool cauliflower and carrots, superb squash, top tomatoes, outstanding onions, radical radishes, lovable leeks, terrific turnips, scrumptious spinach, powerful, pretty peppers etc. Groovy green leafy vegetables like spectacular spinach and groovy green leaf lettuce.

Holy whole grain (breads and cereals).

Radical raw unsalted nuts and seeds like super sunflower seeds, all powerful almonds, wonderful walnuts, etc.

Beautiful beans and beautiful brown rice.

Lovable low-fat yogurt, lovable low-fat cheese, terrific tofu, lovable low-fat milk and low-fat ice cream.

Excellent egg whites (scrambled, hard boiled) or excellent Egg Beaters.

Luscious lean meat, groovy grilled chicken breast, groovy grilled or broiled fish, terrific turkey burgers, vivacious veggie burgers, scrumptious soy burgers.

Happy, healthy oils (like olive, used sparingly in salads).

Super spring water.

Heavenly herbal teas.

It is most important that you focus on eating protein and fiber when you have your meals. Protein takes time to digest and will give you a full feeling compared to carbohydrates and fats. The fiber will also help you feel full by absorbing water and expanding in your stomach. (Talk to your doctor about the many natural fiber supplements available on the market.) Another small thing you can do to get you feeling fuller before you have dinner is to eat a half slice of whole grain bread brushed with pure virgin olive oil. This trick works really well.

It is also important not to go hungry. When you are hungry in between meals and possibly have the urge for a "bad food" snack like chocolate, cookies, or salty chips, wait it out. If you can distract yourself for 10 to 15 minutes, the craving will most definitely go away. If it doesn't, eat a healthy snack first!

Pour a high protein drink over a small serving of high fiber cereal and eat that to make you feel full, or simply eat an apple, some nuts, or low-fat cheese with whole grain crackers. Let healthy food always take care of your hunger! If you have something like low-fat yogurt, low-fat cheese on a whole grain cracker, or a piece of fruit with low-fat cheese before the fattening food, the craving for the bad food should disappear, or at least lessen. If it doesn't, then go ahead and have that tiny taste of chocolate or a tiny teaspoon of that ice cream—or whatever it may be. Keep the amount of that bad food to an absolute minimum and eat it slowly, really enjoying the taste. It's even better to find the least fattening bad food you can find as a substitute. Read labels!

This applies to drinking too. If you really have a craving for a calorie packed sweet drink, have a sip (fill up a shot glass), savoring the taste, then drink a lot of water to quench your thirst. Finally, if necessary, follow with another half or full shot of the calorie-packed drink and savor the taste again. This technique works very well at cutting out unnecessary calories!

And of course, always remember to keep your mind strong and sharp using your affirmations!

Remember, the Good Stuff list is just a general guideline. There are plenty of other healthy foods at the supermarket and your local health food store, as well as natural fiber supplements. Do some research, talk to your doctor, or surf the Internet to see which ones are best for you.

The Bad Stuff

All white flour products such as worthless white bread, loser large bagels, worthless white rice, bad buns, worthless waffles, miserable muffins, pointless pancakes, bad biscuits, pathetic white flour pizza with greasy, fatty cheese, worthless white crackers, worthless white "enriched" pasta, disgusting doughnuts, pathetic pies, crud cookies, etc.

Fatty ice cream, disgusting jellies, frozen yogurt with too many toppings, puddings etc.

Pathetic processed packaged foods (macaroni and cheese) with unhealthy saturated fats and hydrogenated oils

Stupid soda or any stupid sugar-sweetened drinks

Stupid salted snack foods like pathetic potato chips, stupid salted nuts, cruddy white crackers, cheap cheese puffs

Greasy or fried foods

Forgettable, frivolous, fast food, fried food (greasy and salty), disgustingly greasy cheeseburgers, disgustingly greasy fried chicken, bad for you buffalo wings, miserable mozzarella sticks, disgusting, greasy, inedible fries, etc.

The *Affirm & Burn!* philosophy is all about positivity. But if you struggle with the bad foods, here is a sample list of some more negative things you can remember to say or think about them to make them less attractive.

- Full-fat ice cream is chilled fat made for babies and thin, young children. My body is now learning to enjoy superior, healthier, low-fat, alternatives.

• Doughnuts are disgusting, greasy, fatty, man-made, artificial, useless, junk. I have no interest in putting them in my glorious, natural, body. I choose healthier alternatives.

• Soda is disgusting, completely unnatural, acid tasting, corn syrup, man-made, artificial, junk liquid that has no business being in my beautiful, natural body. I now choose to drink beautiful spring water (or club soda) with a splash of natural juice as the perfect, better tasting, better feeling, healthier, happier substitute.

• Processed food with hydrogenated oils are unhealthy and totally unnatural. I avoid them as much as possible.

• Salted, processed, junk, snack foods are a complete waste of time. I don't need them. I don't buy them. I no longer care for them. I now choose and am learning to love eating raw nuts, dried unsulphured fruit, low-fat yogurt or other healthier alternatives.

• Greasy, fried fast food, like French fries, chicken wings, potato skins, and mozzarella sticks, disgust me. It may taste good for a few seconds, but then it makes me miserable and fat for days. I simply do not need that in my life. I avoid it as much as I can.

• Alcohol is unnecessary on my weight loss journey. I may drink a small amount to celebrate after reaching my weight loss goal and then after that only on rare occasions.

Feel free to add to or change the above statements as you see fit. Do whatever works for you, but be realistic and careful not to stress yourself out or develop an eating disorder!

In general, do your best to eat the good stuff whenever possible and refrain from overeating. If at times there is nothing available but the bad stuff, eat as little of it as possible, and always choose to snack on healthy low-fat foods first when you are truly hungry between meals.

Many people will lose weight when they simply eliminate soda or sugary drinks! Others will lose a significant amount of weight when they simply eliminate unhealthy foods like salted snacks (chips, etc.) and sweet snacks (candy, cookies, pastries, etc.) from their diet. This is a very simple thing to do when you use techniques from *Affirm & Burn!*

Remember that the healthier alternatives may not taste as good at first but they will taste better after a certain amount of time. You will get used to them. Don't be like a stubborn child refusing to try new foods. Your body needs just a little time to adjust and learn to like healthier food. Look at it this way: if millions of people can take the time to teach themselves to enjoy horrible tasting things like cigars, cigarettes, and Scotch whiskey, how easy will it be to learn to "acquire a taste" for healthy, natural foods that truly make your body feel better? I will tell you. Very easy!

Another technique to use when you really crave a fattening food and don't want to eat it is to imagine yourself in a swimsuit on a beach looking extremely overweight. See yourself there, looking and feeling horrible as others stare at you. Do whatever you need to do to make this image so painful that you overcome the urge to eat the bad food.

Finally, here's an attitude to have when it comes to willingly not eating pleasurable but fattening foods once you've reached your healthy weight goal. Simply think, "The longer I go without them, the tastier they will be when I finally have them."

For example, if you really loved eating a pint of ice cream with all the fat every night when you were overweight and suddenly you didn't eat ice cream for a week or two, it would taste 10 times as good when you finally did have it! You can do this! Just don't eat the pint! Simply have a tablespoon or two and really savor the taste. The truth, however, of what will probably happen as you get off those fat foods, is that they will no longer appeal to you. Your body will not like it as much. This can only truly be understood through experience so stick with the program and experience it.

If you overeat one day at lunch or dinner don't get upset with yourself. It's not that big a deal. When you do it several days in a row or make it a daily habit is when it becomes a big deal. So if you mess up once in a while, relax and simply eat half portions of healthy food the very next day or two and exercise a little more for a few days to make up for it. *Affirm & Burn!* and be strong!

SIMPLE SAMPLE MENU

Below is a simple sample menu of what you may choose to eat on a daily basis. No one diet is right for everyone. Check with your doctor to see if this works for you and make any changes as necessary.

Breakfast (choose 1, 2, or 3)

1) Have 1/4 cup of steel-cut oatmeal (with some raisins, three or four almonds or walnuts) and/or small serving of low-fat yogurt, water with 1/4 cup unsweetened fruit juice added, or coffee to drink.

2) Make yourself a six-egg white omelette plain or with a cut-up vegetable (pepper, tomato, onion, broccoli, etc.), water with 1/4 cup of unsweetened fruit juice added, or coffee to drink.

3) Have a six-ounce serving of low-fat yogurt with a tablespoon of granola and/or raisins and a few blueberries or raspberries.

Snack

Choose one from the list if you are truly hungry two hours after breakfast. Have your snacks prepared in advance every day!

1) An apple or other fruit with one wedge of low-fat cheese.
2) Small bag of plain or low-calorie flavored popcorn.
3) Handful of sunflower or pumpkin seeds.
4) Palm-sized amount of whole grain crackers.
5) One ounce of high-fiber cereal with a low-calorie, high-protein drink added instead of milk.
6) Rice cake with a thin layer of almond butter spread.

Lunch (choose 1, 2, 3, or 4)

1) Deck of cards-sized amount of grilled chicken with a big green salad complete with lots of veggies and tasty low-fat dressing.
    Water with unsweetened fruit juice added (1/4 cup) to drink.

2) Deck of cards-sized amount of grilled (or canned) salmon with a big green salad complete with lots of veggies and tasty low-fat dressing.
    Water with unsweetened fruit juice added (1/4 cup) to drink.

3) Deck of cards-sized amount of grilled (or canned) tuna with a big green salad complete with lots of veggies and tasty low-fat dressing.
    Water with unsweetened fruit juice added (1/4 cup) to drink.

4) Sliced turkey on whole wheat toast with lettuce and tomato with a big green salad or raw baby carrots on the side. Water with unsweetened fruit juice added (1/4 cup) to drink.

5) Take a whole wheat fiber wrap and fill it with six cooked egg whites, a deck of cards-sized amount of grilled chicken, or tuna with lettuce, tomatoes, peppers, or any other vegetable you like.

Snack
(Choose one if you are truly hungry two hours after lunch)
1) An apple with one wedge of low-fat cheese.
2) Small bag of plain or low-calorie flavored popcorn.
3) Handful of sunflower or pumpkin seeds.
4) Palm-sized amount of whole grain crackers.
5) One ounce of high-fiber cereal with a low-calorie, high-protein drink added instead of milk.
6) Rice cake with a thin layer of almond butter spread.

Dinner (Choose 1, 2,3, or 4)
1) Deck of cards sized amount of grilled chicken, 1/4 cup brown rice, a green leaf salad with tasty low-fat dressing. Water with unsweetened fruit juice added (1/4 cup) to drink.

2) Deck of cards sized amount of grilled steak, a green salad complete with several vegetables and a tasty low-fat dressing, a small (fist sized) baked potato flavored with teaspoon of olive oil and salt.
Water with unsweetened fruit juice added (1/4 cup) to drink.

3) Deck of cards sized amount of grilled steak, 1/4 cup brown rice, with a green salad and colorful vegetables, and tasty low-fat dressing.
Water with unsweetened fruit juice added (1/4 cup) to drink.

4) Have a healthy low-fat, low-calorie, frozen prepared dinner that contains lean protein, and a vegetable.

Snack
(Choose one if you are truly hungry at night but do not eat too close to your bedtime)
1) An apple with one wedge of low-fat cheese.
2) Small bag of plain or low-calorie flavored popcorn.
3) Handful of sunflower or pumpkin seeds.
4) Palm-sized amount of whole grain crackers.
5) 1 oz. of high fiber cereal with high protein drink poured over it.
6) Rice cake with a thin layer of almond butter spread.
7) Any pre-packaged low-calorie, low-fat dessert snack.

CHAPTER 7

How to Exercise

There is so much information available today regarding exercise. People get confused about how long their workout should be and how many times a week they should do it. Of course, before doing any exercise, get a physical from your doctor and find out what is best for you. You can also get plenty of information absolutely free via the Internet, library, or even personal trainers at most gyms. However, if you are uninterested in doing any of that, here is some basic advice followed by a five-day schedule for exercise.

You have probably heard the old saying, "The hardest part is getting started." No saying applies more to exercise than this one. So many times I personally did not feel like exercising but once I started, in just a moment or two I was in "the zone" feeling great. For those of you who are unfamiliar with "the zone," it is a state where your mind is clear and your body is moving and feeling just as you want it to. "The zone" truly is a wonderful feeling that usually happens during an intense or moderately intense aerobic workout.

As you may or may not know, according to the latest research, intense aerobic workouts, not strength training workouts, burn the most calories. Strength training (exercise with weights) is important for overall health, but if you want to burn the most calories, aerobic exercise is key at least during the first few months. Later on, when you hit a plateau and are having trouble losing more weight, you should incorporate strength training.

Avoid the "No pain, no gain!" mentality. *Affirm & Burn!* is totally against this concept. Exercise and pain should never be mentioned in the same sentence! I personally never allow myself to experience any pain at all when I exercise. If I did, I could never do it regularly. Exercise is all about joy to me, which is why I always look forward to it and do it on a regular basis. At times, you could look at me and think I was in pain by the expression on my face during my workout—but in truth, I'm enjoying it!

Train your mind and body to love the idea of exercise and begin slowly. In other words, if you have not exercised in years, before you decide to jog, simply walk. Set easily attainable goals at first. Try walking for just one or two minutes. If that is a struggle for you cut it down to 30 seconds! I'm serious! Your goals at first must be so easy so that you can always outdo yourself. This is what your subconscious mind (little kid in you) loves to do. Trust me. (If you have forgotten how the subconscious mind works, reread that section.) Then, if after walking you feel like jogging, go ahead and jog until you feel like stopping. If that happens, stop, even if it's after only 10 or 20 seconds! Never force or torture yourself unless, of course, you find joy in that! The point is, you must always choose to enjoy every moment of your workout and only work out harder when you really want to. If you can't exercise at a vigorous pace, simply go back to walking. If you are healthy without injuries, you can always walk.

This may sound silly and too slow, but walking is the best way to start. Why? Because the goal is consistency. The idea is to work out consistently for at least a month. That's how you tap into the supreme power of the subconscious mind and form a natural exercise habit. After a month or so, it will get much easier to consistently exercise for longer, more intense periods of time. But at first, you must make it easy and fun to ensure consistency.

The goal is to teach your mind and body that exercise is easy and extremely pleasurable every time you do it. It must be a situation where you always win and do more than what was expected to you. Do this by setting minuscule goals. Why? Because you always feel great when you feel like you've outdone yourself. Why not feel great about exercise every time you do it? Go by how you feel, and choose to enjoy every moment of your exercise. Before long you will be walking and jogging five full minutes, then ten, etc.

Always, always, always have fun and build up at whatever pace feels comfortable. Forget about what "experts" say about heart rates or how long you should exercise in the beginning. Forget about "No pain, no gain!" That mentality can't create consistency and joy in your life! It never lasts, because if you're overweight right now, you are a person who is motivated by pleasure.

Eating is pleasurable so you need to work with the pleasure principle. Make eating healthy food pleasurable (with affirmations) and exercise pleasurable (with affirmations) by having extremely easy goals that you achieve consistently. Don't worry. Take your time. There will be plenty of time to meet those "standards" of the "experts" in the future. You will get there but you must be patient and enjoy yourself along the way! Forget about fast results. Fast results are for people who think they can only feel good after they have gotten results as quickly as possible. That is hogwash. You can always feel good now, no matter what is going on in your life if you choose to do so. Always! That is what *Affirm & Burn!* is all about.

Don't be like the millions of people who punish themselves on a weight loss program and wait to feel good on "that day when they have finally reached their goal weight." That is just silly and never leads to a healthy change in lifestyle. Even if those people do succeed, over 90 percent of them will gain the weight back and more. Don't be like them. Go slow and focus on feeling good all the time while you are getting there. This way you will reach your goal and are more likely to stay there for good.

The days of doing things like trying to kill yourself by jogging a few miles on a hot day and then feeling so sore the next few days are over. Decide your workouts are all about you feeling good, now and forever.

Again the idea is to train the mind and body so that it always wants to exercise because it is easy, fun, pleasurable, and makes you feel like a superstar, amazing, overachiever!

After a few weeks (or a month or two, however long it takes) do your best to meet the standards of the following schedule below. If it takes longer, so what? You will get there! Once again, a person who loses weight in a relatively short period of time and talks about how hard it was will almost certainly gain back all the weight and more in the near future. Believe me. Don't be that person. Take the time to slowly but surely teach your mind and body that exercise is fun, easy, and the key to feeling good all the time. Make it all about pleasure and you are much more likely to keep doing it.

Enjoy! Have fun and use the joy-power words, your favorite affirmations, great music or all of them combined, to give yourself a boost when you need it most.

In time, exercise for you will be just another normal part of "feeling good body maintenance" that will not even require motivation. It will be as natural, normal, and non-negotiable for you as going to the bathroom.

Here is Jerry's story:

Jerry realized the best way to consistently exercise without having to get motivated about it was to treat it like any other necessary bodily function. That is when the idea of "the bathroom workout" was born. Exercise for Jerry suddenly became synonymous with "going to the bathroom," i.e., moving his bowels. In other words, whether he wanted to or not, every day, he had to "go to the bathroom." No self-induced mental motivation was ever needed for this normal bodily function. Some days going to the bathroom was easy, and other days it was more difficult. (Every human being on planet earth can relate to this!) But that never mattered—it simply had to be done. And when he was done, no matter how little progress was made, he always felt better.

This would be the same attitude he would have toward aerobic exercise—the idea that it "had to be done whether it was difficult or not and that he would always feel better afterward." And it was absolutely true! In fact, he began to develop the same exact mindset on the way to a workout as he did when he walked to a bathroom. A sort of "mindless nonchalant movement to a place where something had to automatically be done" without exception.

It never mattered if thoughts like "I don't have time right now" or "I don't feel like it" entered his mind. He would go to the gym or simply start jogging in place at home anyway, the same way thoughts do not matter when one has to move their bowels. You always go to the bathroom no matter what you think about or if you have time, and you always feel better. This became such a powerful life changing philosophy that he has worked out easily and effortlessly on a regular basis for years. Try it yourself!

A SIMPLE FIVE DAY SCHEDULE FOR EXERCISE

On Mondays and Wednesdays:

Power walk (walk fast) or jog at a moderately intense pace for at least 30 to 40 minutes.

Once you become comfortable with that, to burn even more calories, exercise up a hill while carrying some extra weight. For instance, try exercising with 1 lb. to 5 lb. weights in your hands, swinging them with your arms as you walk or jog. Another interesting method is to walk or jog outside while wearing a backpack filled with some hardcover books. Be creative!

Do not, however, strain yourself or do one type of exercise all the time. You should be able to talk during your workout and not desperately gasp for air. If you are at the point where you can't talk, your body will stop burning fat! Be smart!

Always train properly. Do a variety of activities as well during your workouts so you do not get bored or overwork any specific parts of your body. You do not want to cause injury to yourself by overworking the same joints in your body. Mix things up. At the gym or at home, walking outside or on a treadmill is fine, but if you jog, try jogging for 10 minutes and then stop and do as many jumping jacks as you can. After the jumping jacks, get on a bike. Get the idea? Do what you like, be creative, and have fun.

On Tuesdays and Thursdays:

Mix it up! Get on that stair machine, treadmill, elliptical machine, exercise bike, or go outside and walk or jog very lightly as a warmup for five to seven minutes. Then, when you are warm and ready, jog at a more intense pace for 10 to 15 minutes or do some intense jumping jacks. (Use the joy-power words at this time!) Then go back to walking again as a cool-down. This is known as interval training, and it is the best way to train your body to burn calories.

On Saturday or Sunday:

Power walk, hike, jog, dance, jump rope, use an elliptical machine, exercise bike, or stair machine, play a running and chasing game with kids, etc., at a moderate pace for 60 to 95 minutes at least once a week. The idea is to do something active that you can enjoy for more than an hour.

For instance, if you have some shopping to do at the mall, park as far away from the entrance as possible. Then walk completely around the outside of the mall once or twice before going in. Once you are in, walk throughout the entire mall at a moderate pace observing everything before you go into any store and do any shopping. Sure, people might stare at you, but who cares? You're burning calories and getting lighter!

That's about it. Exercise is not that complicated. It's all about breathing, moving and getting that blood pumping. If you want more information search the Internet (there is so much fantastic and absolutely free information available there!) or go to a library or bookstore and check out dozens of books or magazines on the subject! You can also get plenty of ideas from trainers at any gym in your area. Information about exercise is everywhere and most often absolutely free.

If you are a busy stay-at-home parent with little time to exercise, arrange to exercise with your kids during the day. Spend 10 to 20 minutes dancing, doing jumping jacks, or whatever to some of your favorite songs. The kids will love it and fall asleep much faster at night. You will too!

Exercise never has to be boring. Music is an excellent way to make it fun. Invest in a portable music-playing device if you haven't already. They are worth their weight in gold!

CHAPTER 8

THE HEALTH CEREMONY

You played with the affirmations and rhymes ("dating"). You started to notice them working after a short time and began to get more serious about them ("engaged"). You've been eating healthier and exercising and feeling good as a result. You realized you liked what was happening and wanted to become fully committed to a healthy lifestyle. You are now ready to plan a Health Ceremony ("wedding"), which can also be called a symbolic "marriage of the mind and the body."

What exactly is a Health Ceremony?

A Health Ceremony is like a wedding ceremony, only much more important. It is a ceremony showing your commitment to living a healthier lifestyle. When you are committed to living a healthier lifestyle (eating healthier foods and exercising), you will feel better. When you feel better, it is easier to get along with others and life becomes more joyful. Always remember that committing to your own mind/body health is as much as a gift to others as it is to you.

Why have a Health Ceremony?

Ceremonies or rituals have existed among human beings from all cultures for thousands of years. Today we have ceremonies for numerous occasions: weddings, graduations, career promotions, etc. Nearly all religions use ceremonies to emphasize a change of life. For example, Christians have a confirmation and Jews have a bar mitzvah. They are spiritual events that affect us in ways we do not always consciously understand. The truth is they affect the deeper part of our mind (the subconscious "little kid in you"), which is crucial when you want to make lasting changes in your life. A special ceremony like the Health Ceremony will make the impression on your subconscious, that "getting healthy is a good thing with no negative consequences."

Too many people have forgotten the true purpose and meaning of a sacred ceremony. That is why one is needed now more than ever. In a sense, your Health Ceremony is you saying goodbye to your careless lifestyle of eating any food, good or bad, as much as you want without considering the consequences. This is similar to the bachelor/bachelorette who, before his/her wedding must say goodbye to their careless past and all the bad relationships with others. All ceremonies/rituals are beautiful but serious spiritual events. They help solidify the commitment to personal growth.

Even if you don't understand how the subconscious works, the good news is it doesn't matter. That's right—it does not matter! Your subconscious will get it. Just have the Health Ceremony and realize that it is a positive thing and part of the easy way of "putting you on autopilot" toward reaching your health goal.

In general, your Health Ceremony will be very similar to a wedding ceremony, so you may simply use what happens at a wedding ceremony as a basic guideline. You can do it with a group of friends or make it very personal and do it alone, whatever is most comfortable for you. There are no set rules, but here is a basic guideline as to how you could do it.

Before you start you will need:
1) a music player (to play soothing music)
2) candle(s) and matches
3) incense

4) a ring

5) a clay model molded to look like your body and a
   small plastic knife, or a pencil drawing of your body
   on paper, or a photo of yourself along with a photo of
   your goal body (get this from a magazine or the Internet)

6) a comfortable place to lie down

7) your top 10 affirmations

The ceremony should start at a specific time with soothing music. You should be dressed in something special (your best exercise outfit would be appropriate). It can take place indoors or outdoors. It is up to you. What is most important is that it be an enjoyable but serious event that has special meaning to you. It should generate emotion and inspiring words should be said, just like a wedding.

Start by lighting a candle and then having someone or yourself read the statement below.

Dearly beloved. We are gathered here today to become aware and pledge our undying loyalty to our closest and best friend; the part of us that has been with us since birth and will never leave us until the day we die, and truly the first and most loyal friend we will ever have—our body. We begin this ceremony by first saying with the utmost sincerity (repeat after me) "I am sorry, body, for not taking care of you the way I should have. I am sorry for overfeeding you and giving you foods or other substances that did not truly nourish you.

I am sorry that you have had to work harder than you should have all this time due to the extra weight I put on you. I am truly sorry and I know that you truly forgive me and are on my side willing to work with me to make you stronger, lighter, and healthier. From this day on I will choose to live a healthy lifestyle not because I or others think I should, but because I now know that this is the first essential step to true lasting happiness."

Look at your clay model, drawing, or photo. Say, *"I know a lighter, healthier, person is inside this body waiting to emerge. I will succeed in creating this lighter, healthier body."*

Peel off enough clay (with your knife or hands) to reveal the kind of body you want, erase your drawing and redraw yourself with the kind of body you desire, or look at the photo of your goal body.

Say, *"How do I know a lighter, healthier, person is inside this body waiting to emerge and that I will succeed in creating this lighter, healthier body? Because..."*

(Play soothing music) Read your top 20 affirmations slowly and with feeling. Repeat any specific affirmations more than once if you like. When you are done you may put on your ring at this time if you like—wearing a ring or bracelet as a symbol of your commitment is up to you. Now, find a comfortable spot to lie down. Close your eyes, and use soothing music and incense to get yourself into a relaxed state. In this state visualize all the parts of your body relaxing starting at the bottom and working your way to the top. Thank each body part too. Start out with the basics, relaxing and thanking your toes, feet, ankles, calf muscle, knees, etc. for working as best they could for you. And then include everything about your body you can think of internally (bones, blood, arteries, veins, organs). Relax and enjoy this process.

Then, imagine a large sphere of healing light enveloping you from head to toe. It can be any color you want—white, bluish white, green, violet, yellow—whatever suits you. See this light as a healing to your body. Stay in this relaxed state for as long as you like and then visualize yourself looking at your body in a mirror the way you want it to look. Make this image as real as possible! Spend as much time as you need to do this. This will be the image you can recall during those times you are tempted to go off your health regime. When you open your eyes the ceremony is over.

If you have trouble visualizing you can cut out an ideal body picture for yourself from a magazine or from the Internet, paste a photo of your head on to it and use that. Keep this picture in your wallet so you will always have it with you. Make several of them with different outfits if you like. Be creative and have fun.

In general, make your ritual memorable and something you look forward to doing. You can add more or skip whatever parts you want in the above example. It is up to you. Make it fun! You should, however, renew your vows and repeat this ceremony (especially the visualizing) in a shortened form at least once a week, the way many people attend a church or temple at least once a week. Ultimately there are no rules as long as everything is positive and leads you toward your health goal!

Right After the Health Ceremony (or the very next day):

1. Go to your refrigerator, food cabinet, car, work cubicle, and any other place where there is fattening, unnecessary, unhealthy, food, like cookies, potato chips, donuts, candy, cakes, ice cream, etc., and throw them away. No exceptions! No thinking about it, no considering, no excuses. Throw it away! You can't eat what is not there.

This sounds depressing, but it isn't. It is extremely important and very liberating. Getting rid of your useless garbage is empowering! You are leaving that junk behind and creating a stronger, healthier, happier life. Like a drug addict throwing away all their drugs or an alcoholic getting rid of all the alcohol in the house, you must do this. You do not need those junk foods any more! They harm your body just as alcohol and drugs harm the body and you are choosing to stop this. This is an essential part of your decision to win no matter what happens.

And by the way, if you think it's wrong to throw away fattening food because there are starving people in the world, other people in your house who can eat it, or people at work that enjoy that food who don't have a weight problem, think again. It's not wrong. It's junk food!

Make everyone aware of a new rule that will take effect as you begin your new healthy lifestyle. If those people want their unhealthy, fattening food then they need to keep it hidden under lock and key away from you. They are not allowed to eat it in front of you. No exceptions! If you see that fattening food, tell them it will be crushed and thrown away. It does not matter how much food or money is wasted; it will be crushed and thrown away. You will replace these horrible "foods" with healthy foods from the good list. Fruits and other healthy snacks like low-fat yogurt, low-fat cheese, cottage cheese, vegetables, raw nuts, seeds, whole grain crackers, etc., will take their place!

Getting rid of all the fattening snack food in your home is important, especially if you have trouble at night. This is true for so many people. It is so easy to eat the wrong things at night if you become lonely, bored, or a little depressed. These wrong foods almost become like "old silent friends" you have always counted on. It can feel as if they have always been there and have never let you down and you can get sad that they are not around and you can't enjoy them. This is understandable and I think at some point there isn't anyone who can say they have not struggled with this at times. That is why these fattening foods simply can't be in the house!

So what to do if you are sad at night and really, really want to eat a bag of potato chips, cookies, candy, or ice cream, and you just might even get dressed and go to a store to get it? Don't do it! Be sad. Yes, be sad. Accept that sad emotion and go to bed. Then, while you're in bed, read the parts of *Affirm & Burn!* that will remind you of what you're doing. When you wake, you are going to feel so good as you congratulate yourself for doing what you knew was right the night before! Believe me: you lost more fat off your body because you didn't give in to your temptation! Congratulate yourself many, many times in the morning. Also be sure to repeat an appropriate affirmation in the morning that makes you feel really good about your accomplishment the night before!

One last thing: It is also important to declutter your house and workplace after your Health Ceremony. Throw out all the useless junk (old clothing, etc.), that you have been saving for no reason. You know what I'm talking about! If it has not been used in over a year, let it go! Sell it, give it to charity, or throw it away. This will help with your weight loss goal. It will feel as if your house and/or workplace lost weight too and you will feel so much better about yourself as well. Trust me. Do it!

CHAPTER 9

Simple Summary for Affirm & Burn!

• Decide getting lighter and healthy is something you absolutely want to do and go for it 100 percent with a totally positive attitude. No exceptions! DECIDE! This is not a difficult decision! Refuse to say or think anything negative about eating healthy or exercising and have a completely open mind as you follow the *Affirm & Burn!* philosophy.

• Read everything again, in its entirety (don't do anything until you've read it all again), and then go back to the beginning and follow the instructions. For the first two weeks just "play," saying your affirmations daily. The focus should be totally on the mind and "feeding" it constantly with the awesome affirmations. Do not cheat by forcing yourself to actually eat healthier or exercise at all at this time unless you truly feel the desire to. *Affirm & Burn!* is designed to get your mind in shape first so your weight loss journey becomes a pleasurable process. Suffering is not a part of the program. Suffering can only happen in the mind and if your mind is right there will be no suffering during your health program. All you are really required to do at this point is to keep an open mind, play and have fun by reading all the affirms that "click" with you. Read and repeat them often with conviction throughout your day especially in the morning and before you go to sleep. (It takes less than five minutes to do this and it is easy and fun. If you can read all of the added material in *Affirm & Burn!* that is great too!)

• In addition you will post two or more of your favorite affirmations in your bedroom, bathroom and anywhere else in your environment where you can see and read them often (with feeling, out loud or in your mind). Reading them first thing in the morning is especially important because that is when your mind is most open to suggestion. Also keep in mind that the more you "get a little crazy" with this by covering the walls of your environment with affirmations and repeating them throughout the day, the easier it will be for you to transform yourself into a lighter, healthier, person. Repetition with feeling is key! Getting crazy about being light and healthy is a good thing at the start of your program!

Of course everyone has their obligations, so do the best you can. At the very least, get into the habit of repeating an affirmation multiple times when you do things you must do every day, such as waking up, going to the bathroom, getting showered, brushing your teeth, getting dressed, just before you eat or exercise, and every time you are in a bathroom during the day.

• It is also fun and effective to memorize at least one of your favorite rhyme affirmations and say (or sing) it with feeling throughout your day. Just one rhyme affirmation may be all you need to make incredibly positive changes in your life! Just one can work magic for you.

• After a couple of weeks (it might be one week, maybe three— everyone is different and it all depends on how committed you are to repeating your affirms with conviction) the affirms should be affecting your mind and actions. In other words, you will be wanting to eat healthy and exercise as if you have hypnotized yourself. This is an exciting time! You will know it when it is happening. A transformation is taking place. You are becoming a person that desires healthy food and exercise instead of "struggling or feeling like you should." Start eating healthy and exercising and continue affirming as usual! You have found the easy way! When you have been eating healthy, exercising, and feeling good about it for at least two weeks, it will then be time for your Health Ceremony.

• You will have a Health Ceremony when you have reached the point where eating healthy and exercising feels good and natural for you and you really want to commit even more to it. A Health Ceremony is like a wedding ceremony where you vow to be totally committed to leading a healthy lifestyle. Think of the Health Ceremony as "sealing the deal," and locking yourself into a lifetime of being light and healthy, feeling good, and truly living happily ever after with your body. Live like you're on that magical island where only healthy food exists and exercising is a joy. Never leave that island in your mind! After the ceremony, follow up with a house and workplace cleansing of all junk food, replacing it with healthy alternatives. You can't eat junk if it's not there! Do a pleasant shortened version of the ceremony once a week and scrape a thin layer of clay off of your clay body, or erase and redraw the body you have to the body you want, to symbolize the weight you are losing. Keep it fun, simple, inspiring, and always pleasurable.

• Use the joy-power words (with music if you prefer) and empowering questions, etc., any time you are feeling depressed, lazy, or when you "hit the wall" during a workout. They are also excellent for interval training.

• Continue repeating your affirmations every day. Change them as you see fit. If you are struggling with your eating habits, focus more on the eating affirmations. If people trying to sabotage you is a problem, focus on those affirmations. And so on. Most importantly, enjoy the process! Make everything joyful so it can become a natural way of life for you.

CHAPTER 10

A Final Note

Losing weight is not an impossible task. Millions of people who have struggled with weight loss have actually lost weight many times. The real issue is keeping the weight off and maintaining a healthy lifestyle. The ability to do this is easy when you keep your mind focused on having your body and mind feel good through proper eating and exercise.

Always remember that what you ultimately want in every moment is to feel good or be happy. That's it! And the key to that is eating healthy food in proper portions, exercising on a regular basis, and staying positive. Simply choose to no longer fall into the routine of feeling bad about yourself, overeating for days, weeks, or months, gaining weight, and then punishing yourself once again on a "die"t. Just read and follow the *Affirm & Burn!* philosophy as often as you can (keep those affirmations around) and without trying, your mind will be conditioned to keep you light and healthy.

Remember, when you reach your goal weight, it's not similar to reaching any other simple goal, like passing your driving test or graduating from a school. You don't you get that official paper that says, "You are officially done for the rest of your life!" After you reach a weight loss goal you still must pay attention or you will gain the weight back.

Accomplishing your weight loss goal is nothing like getting a diploma from a school because when you get a diploma you don't have to pay attention anymore. You can be lazy and forget everything you ever learned in school and they won't take your diploma away! It is yours forever.

With weight loss, however, it is a different story. The weight can easily come back. You can "lose your diploma!" So you must pay attention. If you stop paying attention and get a little lazy, a few pounds a week will creep on to your body and after a short time, you can be overweight again. Don't let this happen to you. If it does, deal with the problem quickly. Remind yourself that life is about feeling good and if you are putting on weight, you're making food too much of your "feel good formula " in life.

Decide that if you get off track you will never let yourself gain more than three to five pounds. Ever! If you do—*Affirm & Burn!* Immediately go back to eating healthy and exercising and keep your mind filled with empowering thoughts! Vow to be alert and aware so those pounds don't come back!

It's not that you get off track; we all do. It's how long you get off track. Never, ever, ever allow yourself to get off track too long! If this happens, be sure to focus your mind once again on proper eating and exercise and always—

AFFIRM & BURN!

On the following pages are some of the more popular affirmations with photos (and some health ads) that you can print or screenshot when you need more inspiration. Feel free to find photos that you like and create your own.

Chapter 11
Bonus Photos

Empowering Ads

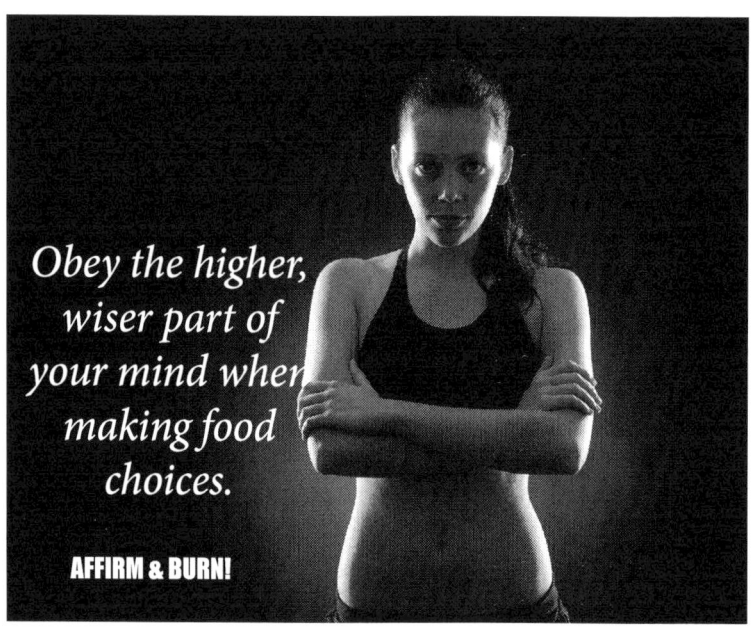

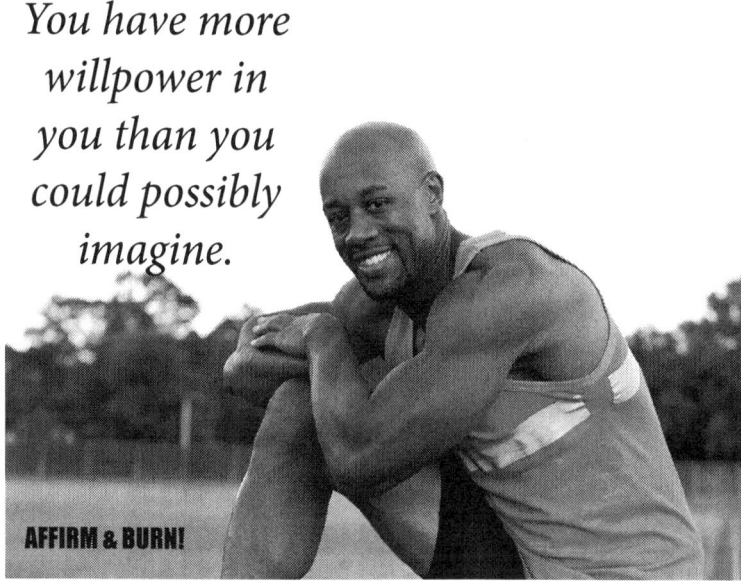

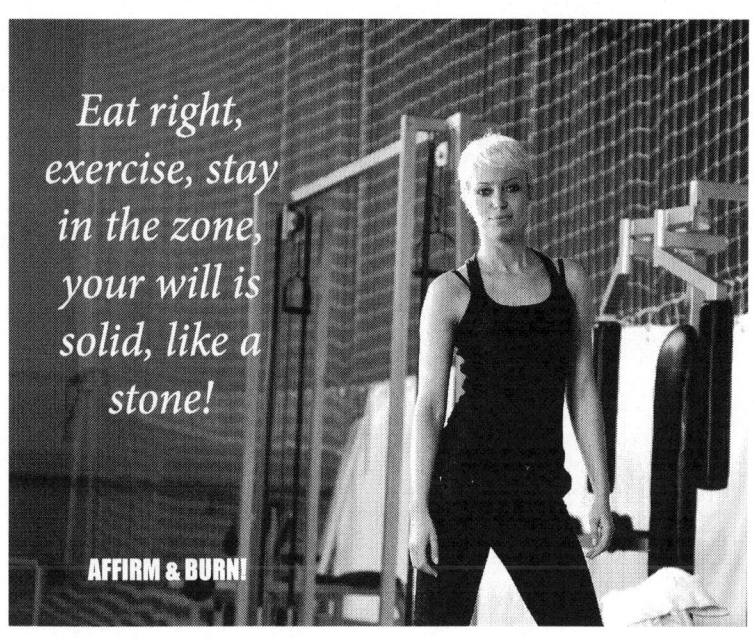

Eat right, exercise, stay in the zone, your will is solid, like a stone!

AFFIRM & BURN!

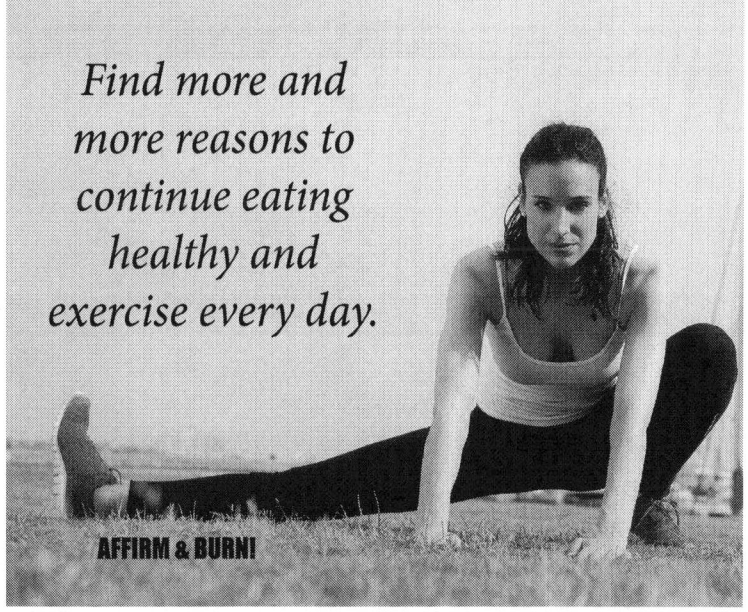

Find more and more reasons to continue eating healthy and exercise every day.

AFFIRM & BURN!

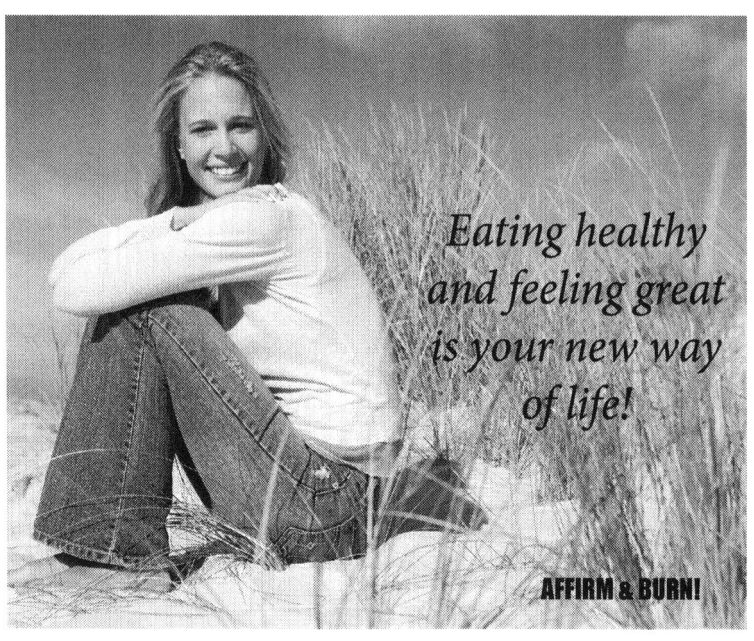

Eating healthy and feeling great is your new way of life!

AFFIRM & BURN!

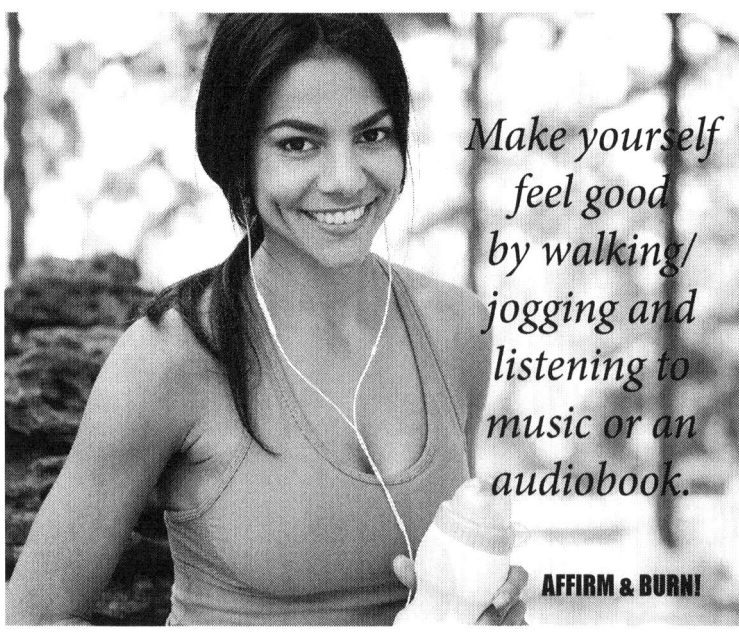

Make yourself feel good by walking/ jogging and listening to music or an audiobook.

AFFIRM & BURN!

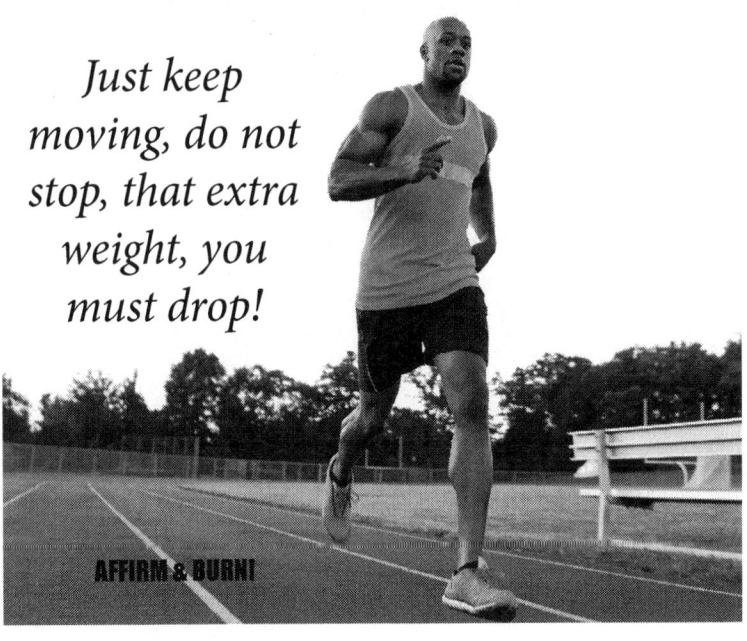

Just keep moving, do not stop, that extra weight, you must drop!

AFFIRM & BURN!

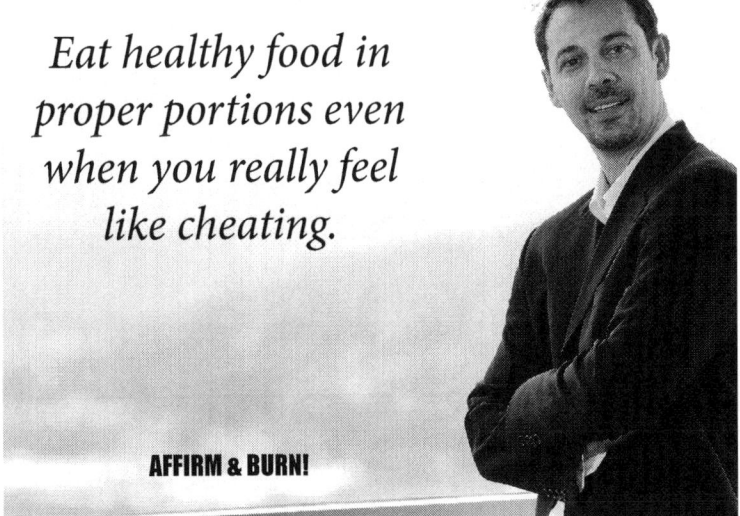

Eat healthy food in proper portions even when you really feel like cheating.

AFFIRM & BURN!

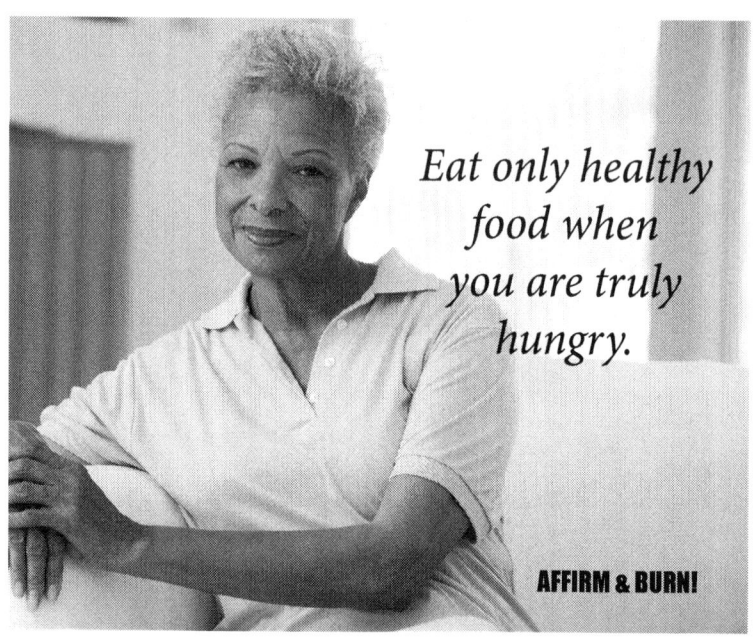

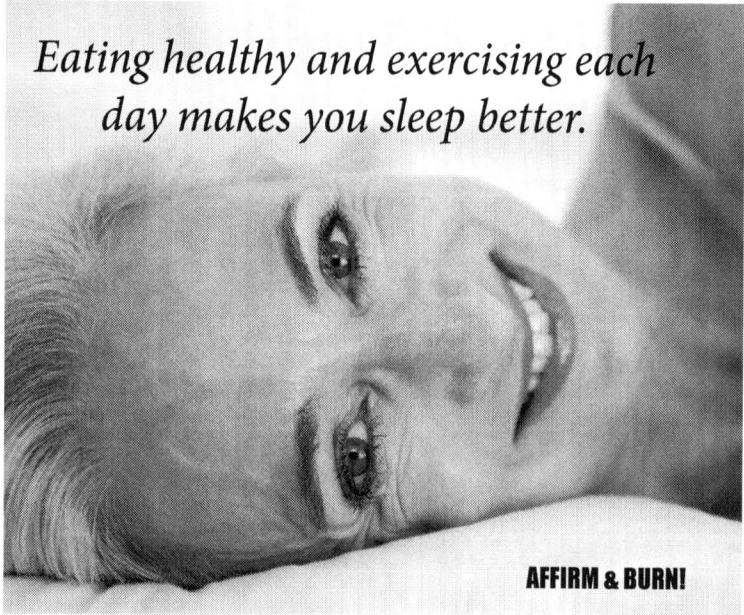

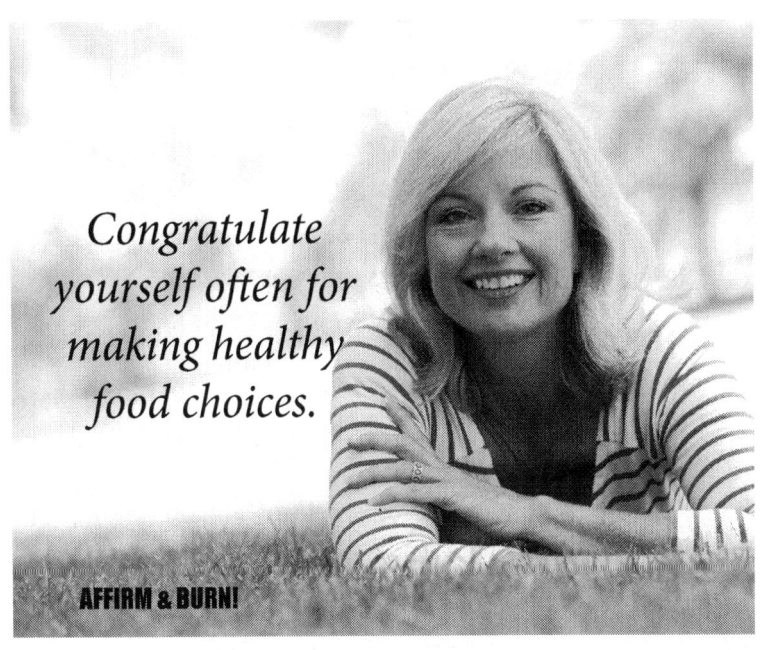

Congratulate yourself often for making healthy food choices.

AFFIRM & BURN!

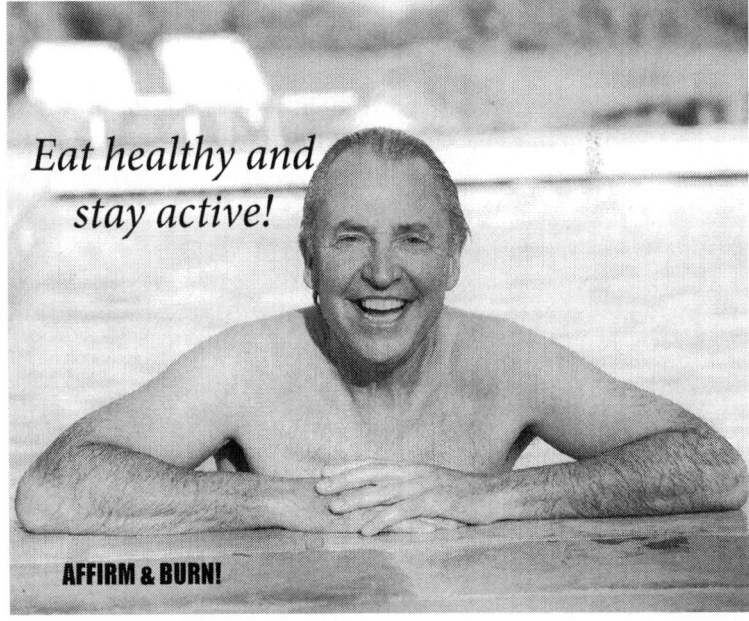

Eat healthy and stay active!

AFFIRM & BURN!

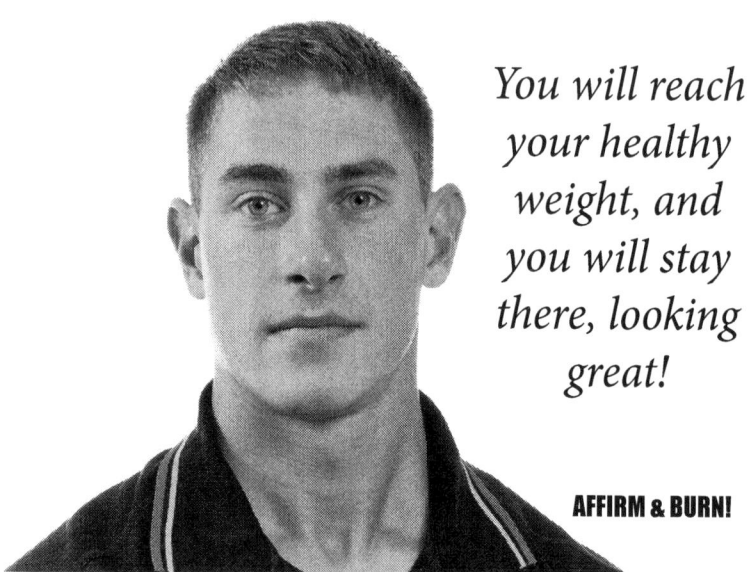

*You will reach
your healthy
weight, and
you will stay
there, looking
great!*

AFFIRM & BURN!

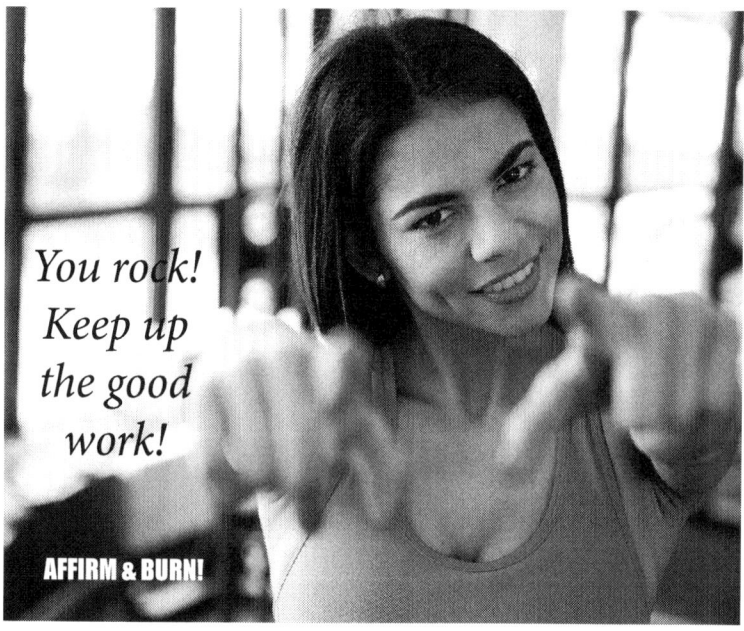

*You rock!
Keep up
the good
work!*

AFFIRM & BURN!

THE RHYMES

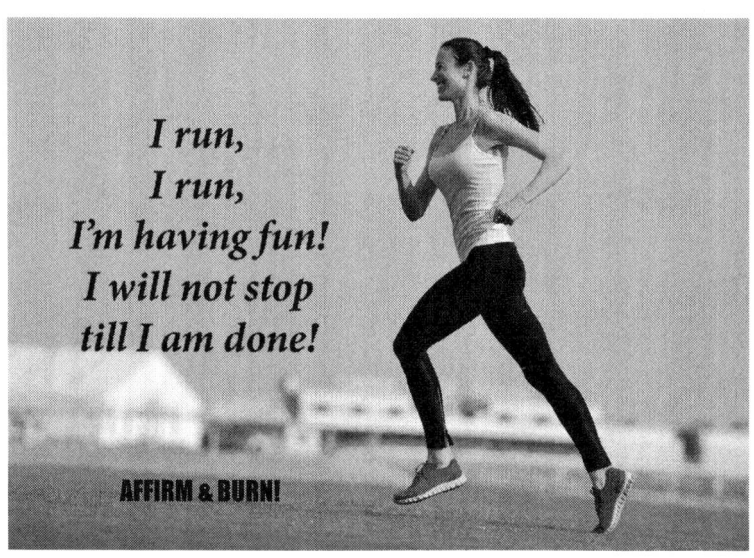

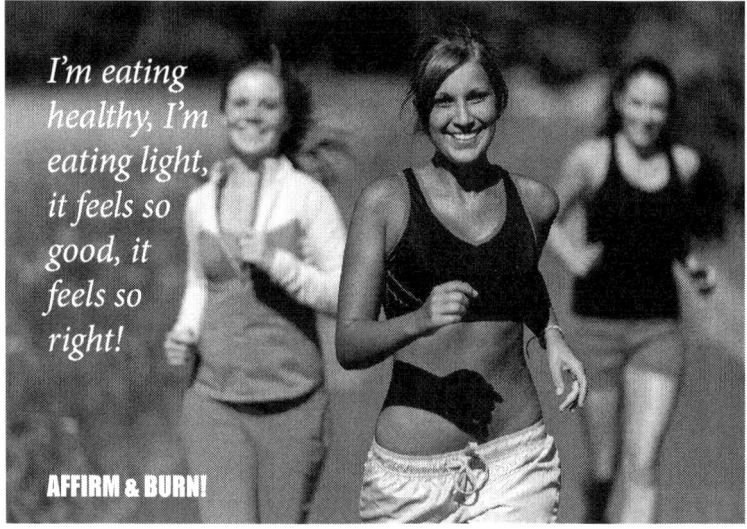

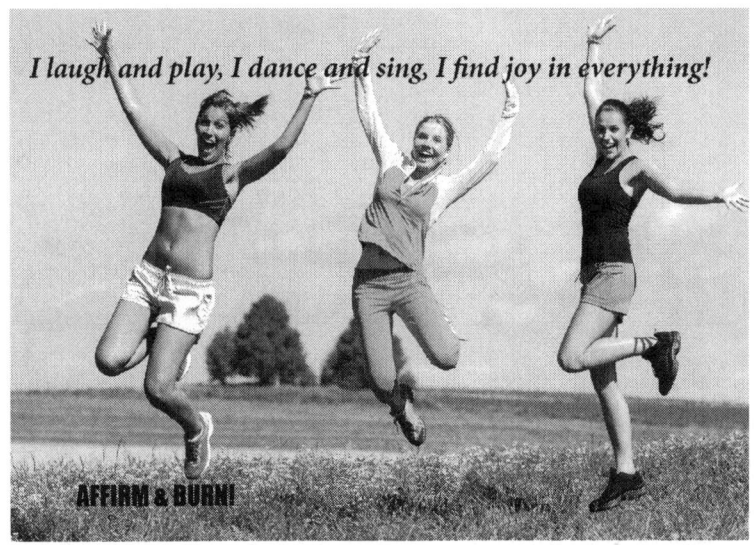

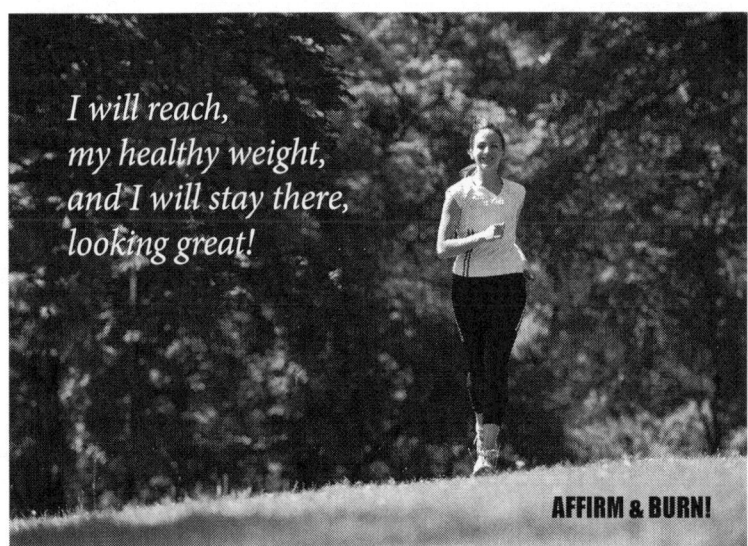

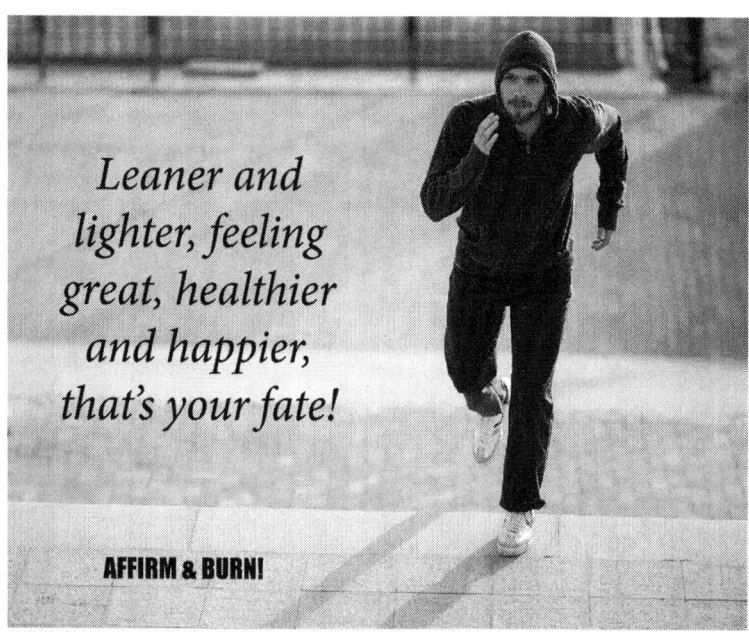

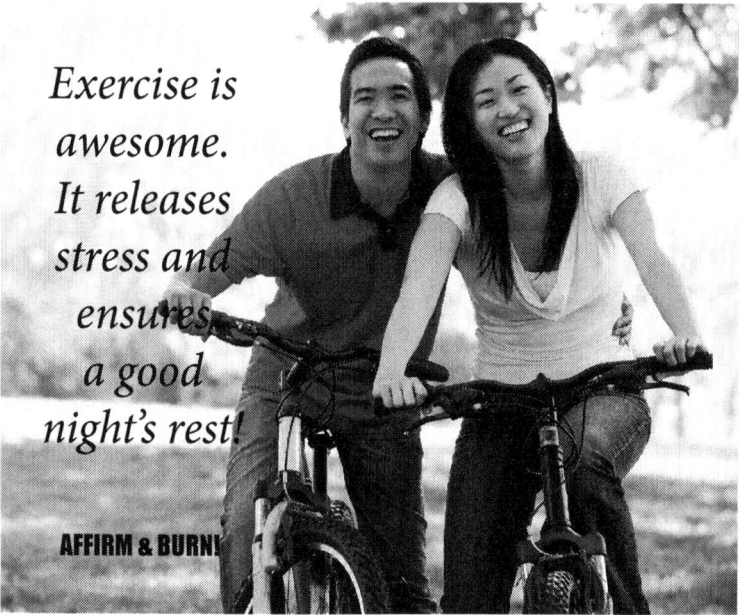

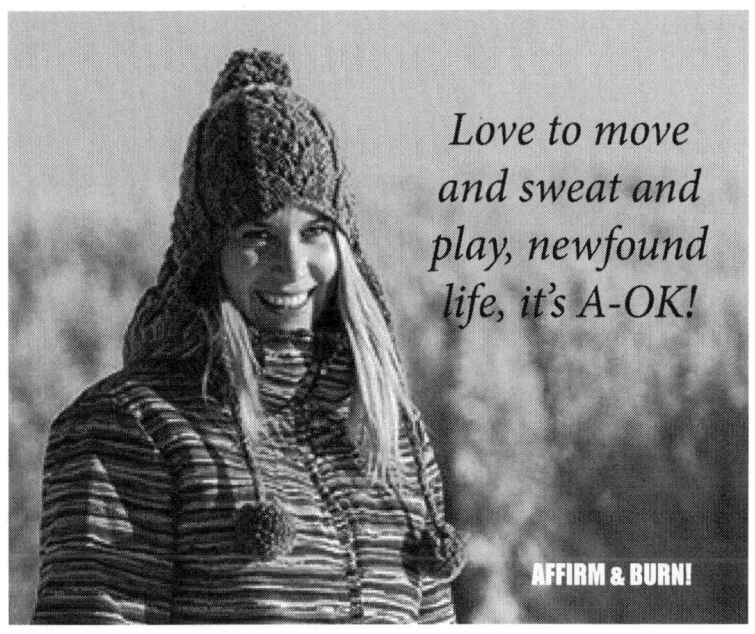

Love to move and sweat and play, newfound life, it's A-OK!

AFFIRM & BURN!

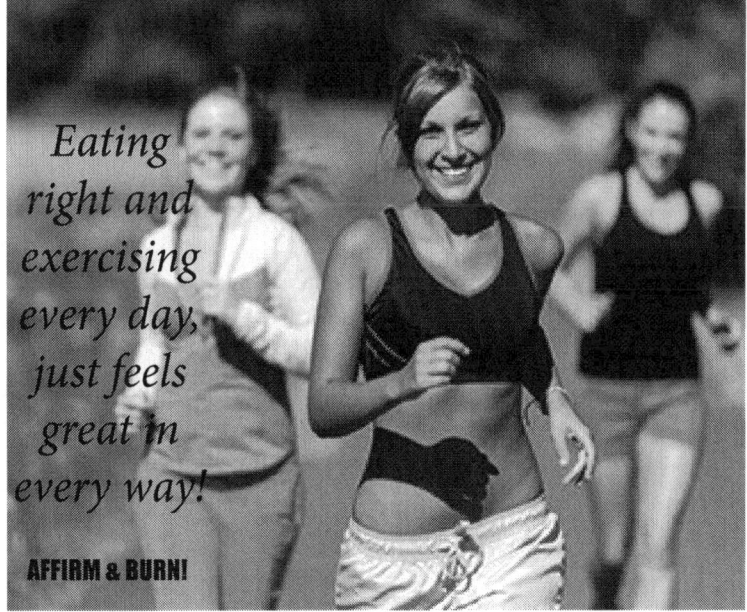

Eating right and exercising every day, just feels great in every way!

AFFIRM & BURN!

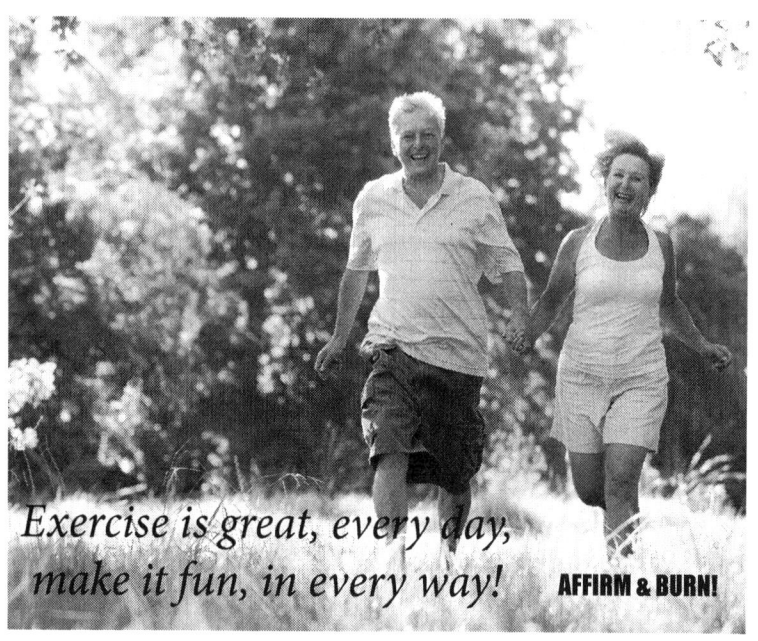

Exercise is great, every day, make it fun, in every way! **AFFIRM & BURN!**

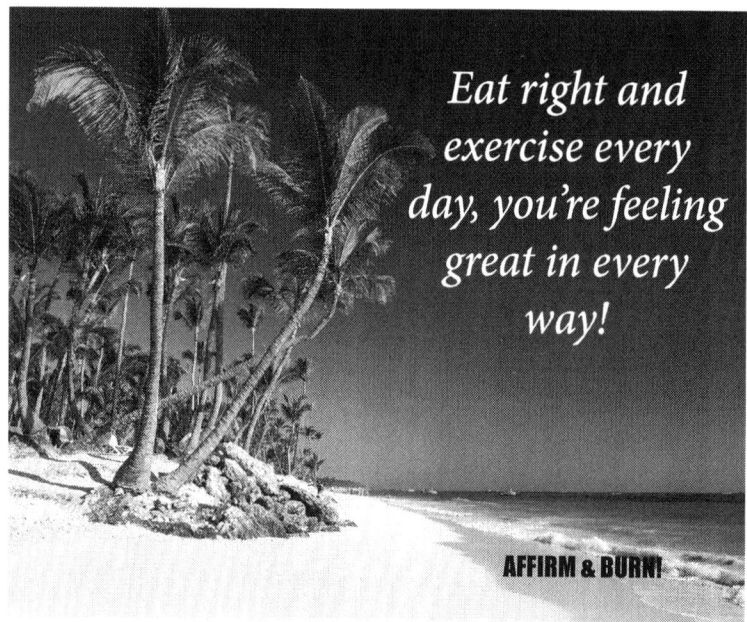

Eat right and exercise every day, you're feeling great in every way!

AFFIRM & BURN!

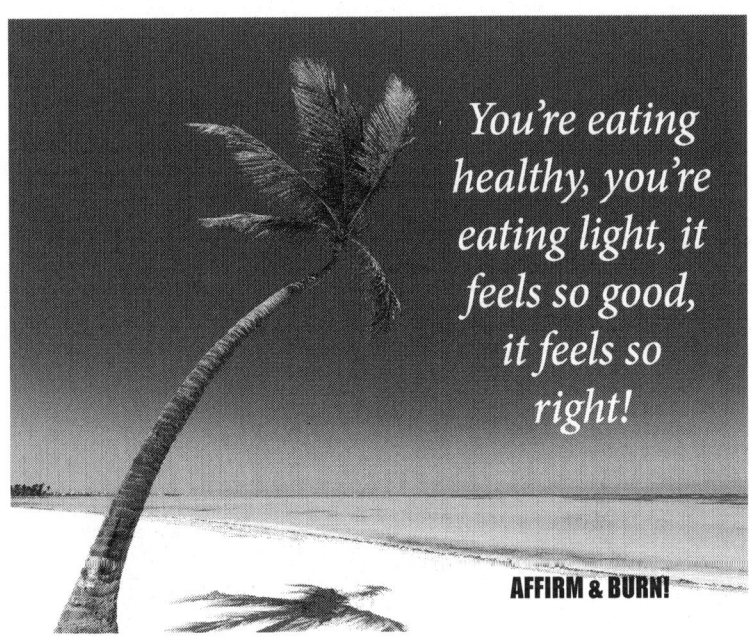

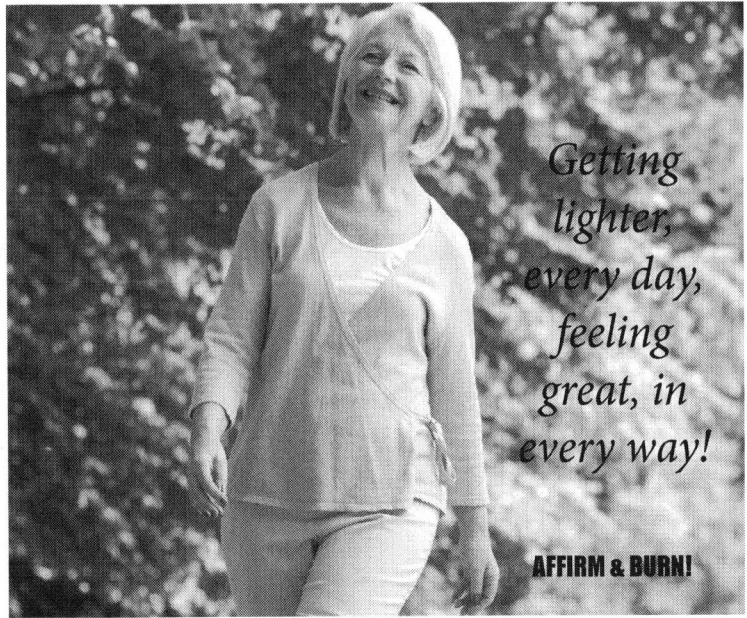

FOOD ADS

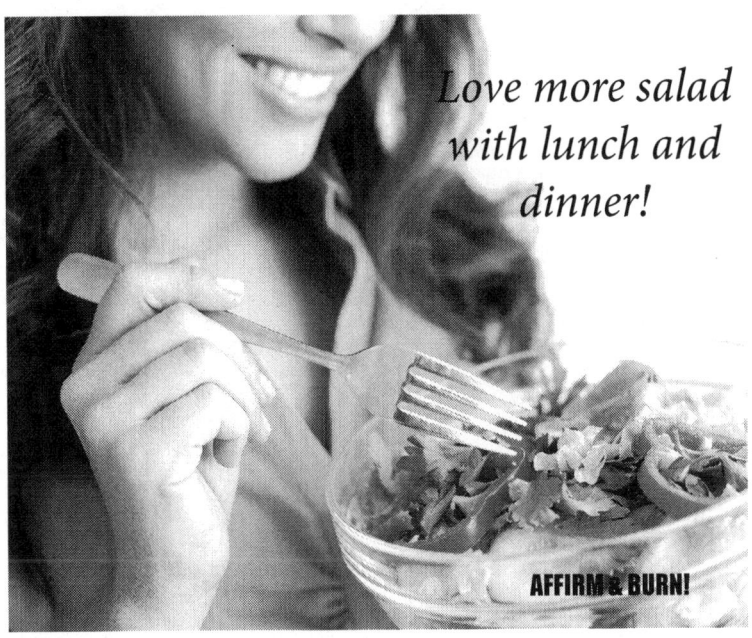

Love more salad with lunch and dinner!

AFFIRM & BURN!

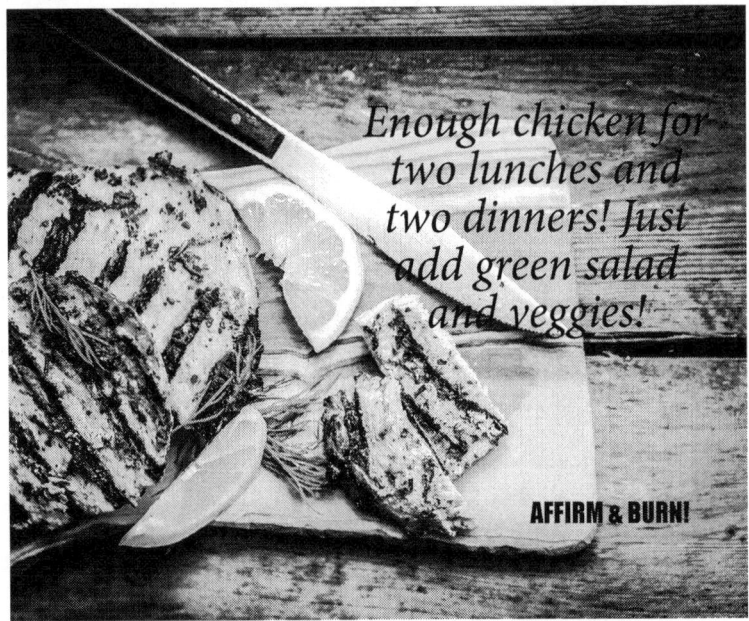

Enough chicken for two lunches and two dinners! Just add green salad and veggies!

AFFIRM & BURN!

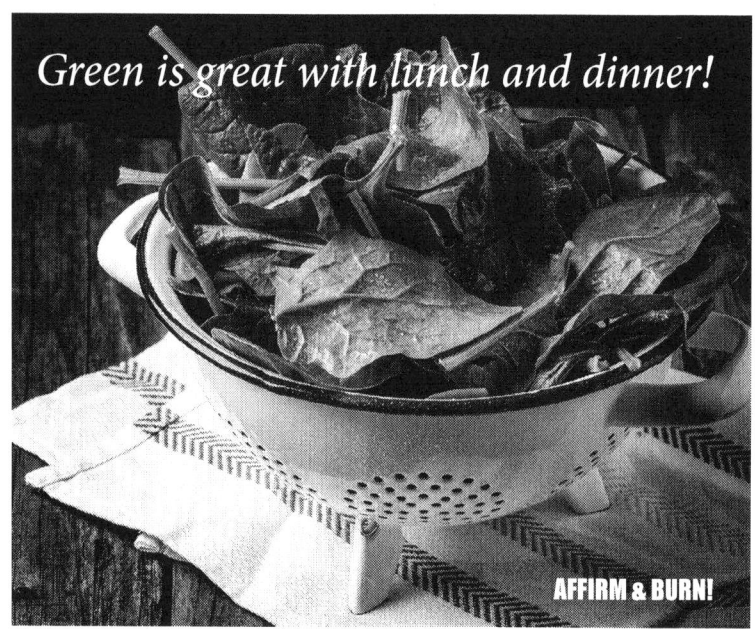

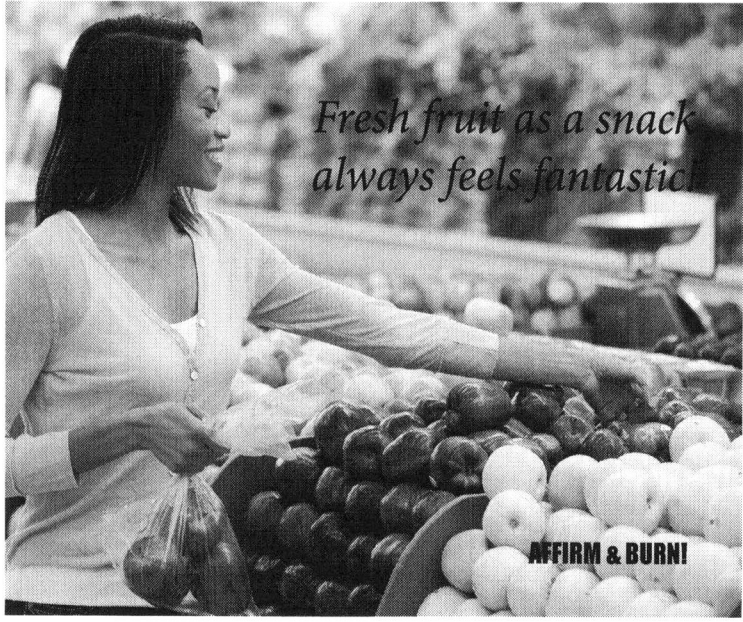

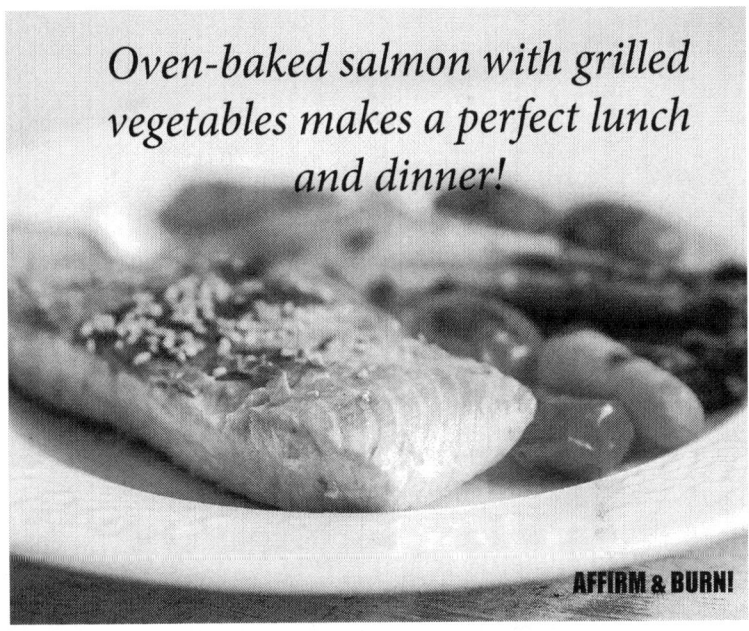

Oven-baked salmon with grilled vegetables makes a perfect lunch and dinner!

AFFIRM & BURN!

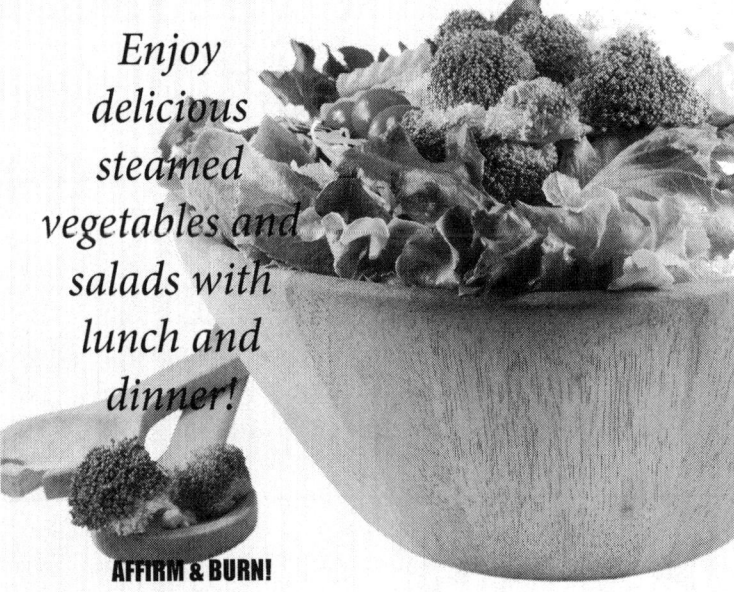

Enjoy delicious steamed vegetables and salads with lunch and dinner!

AFFIRM & BURN!

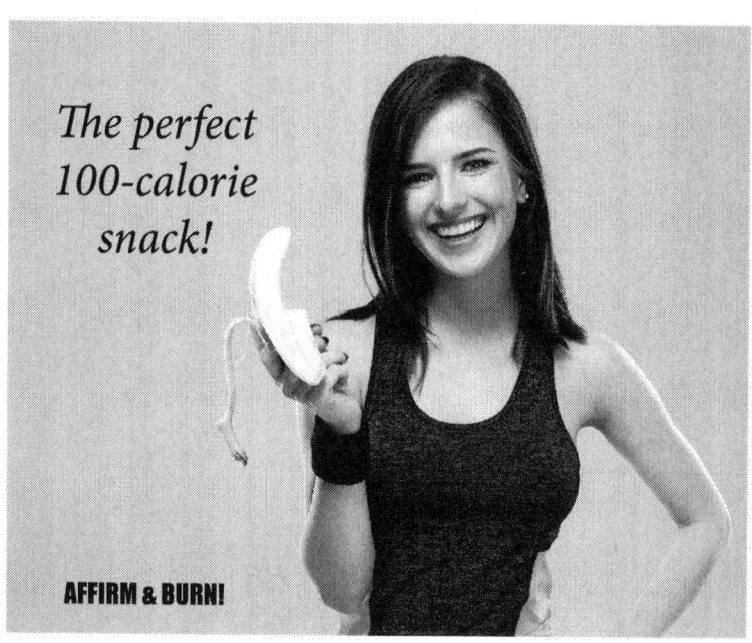

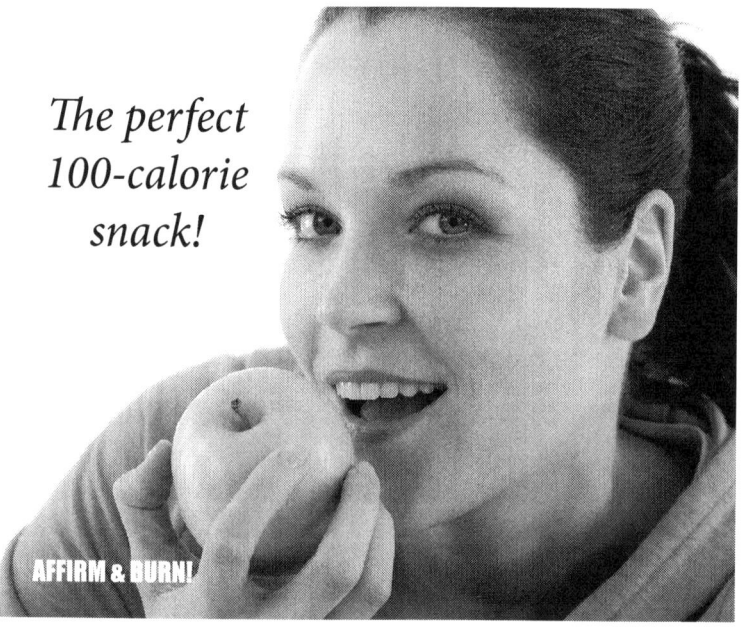

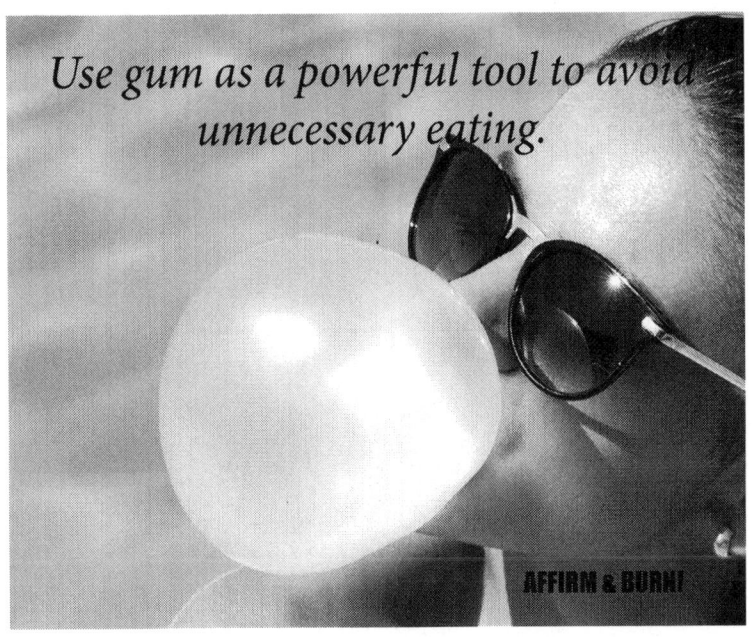

Use gum as a powerful tool to avoid unnecessary eating.

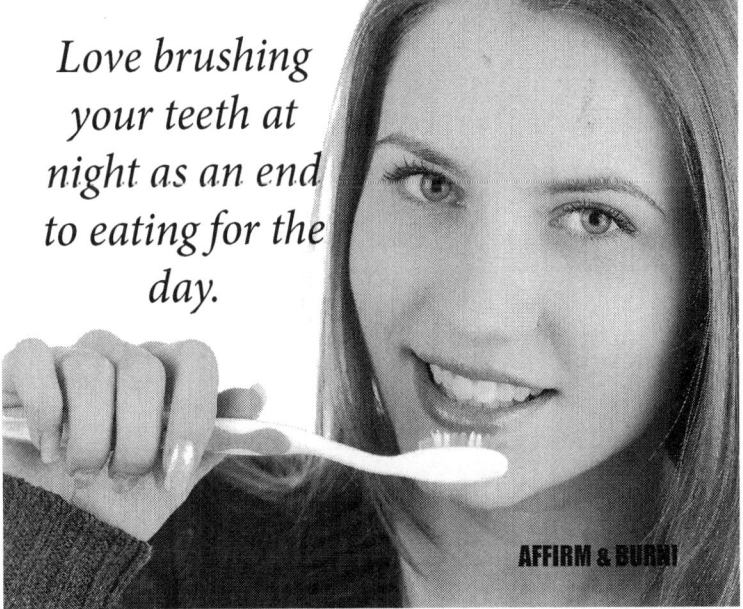

Love brushing your teeth at night as an end to eating for the day.

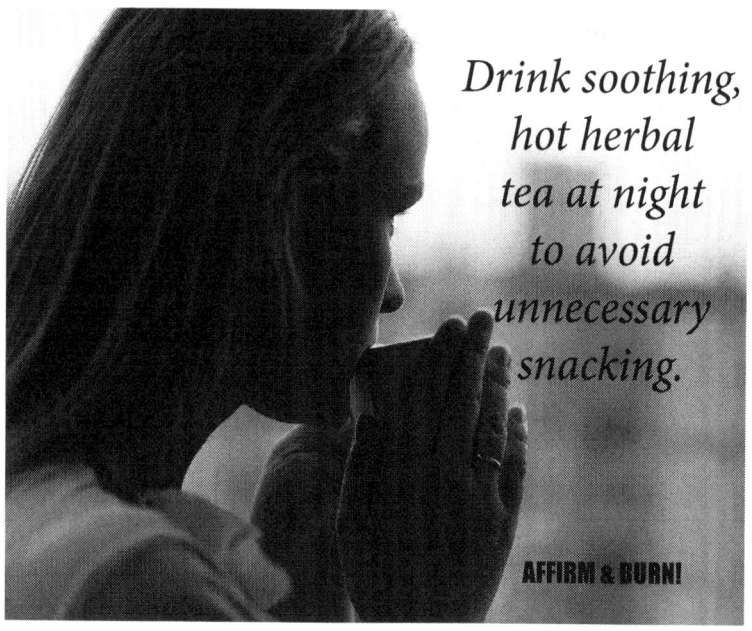

Drink soothing, hot herbal tea at night to avoid unnecessary snacking.

AFFIRM & BURN!

AFFIRMATION ADS

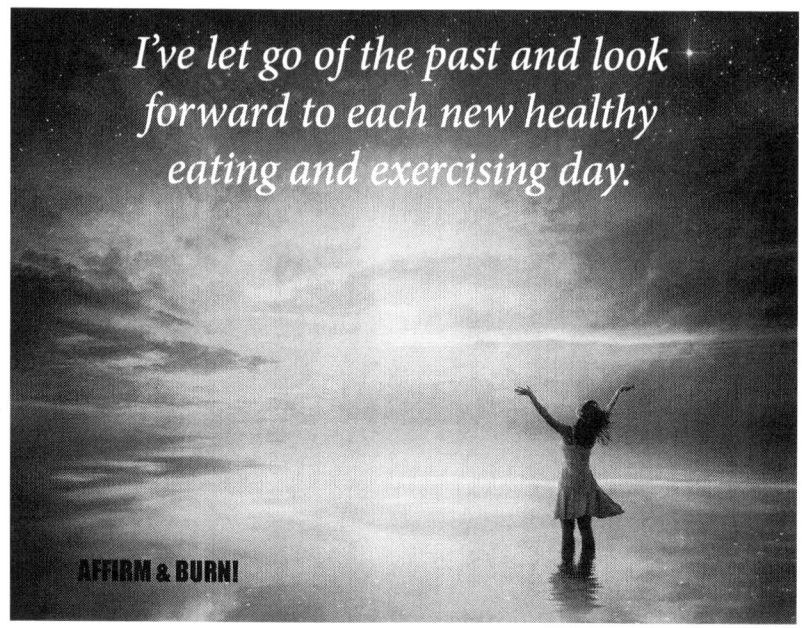

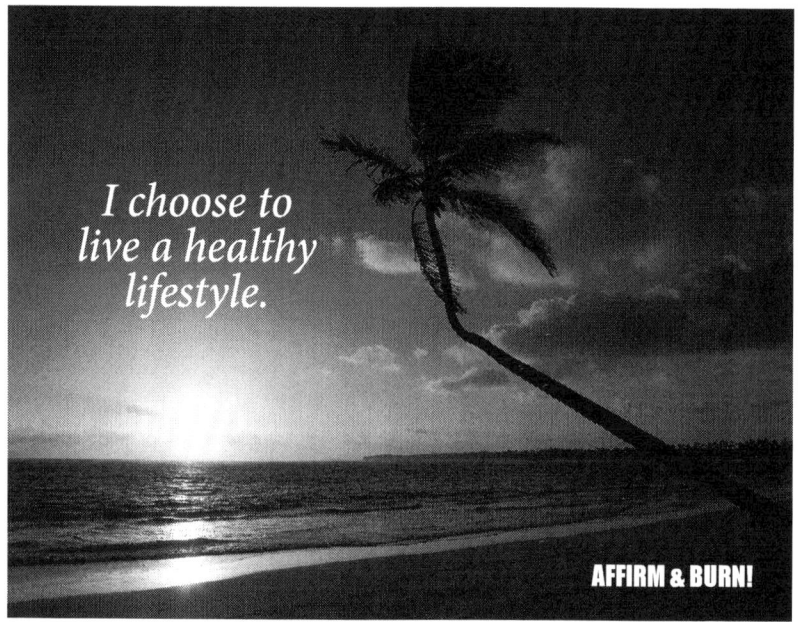

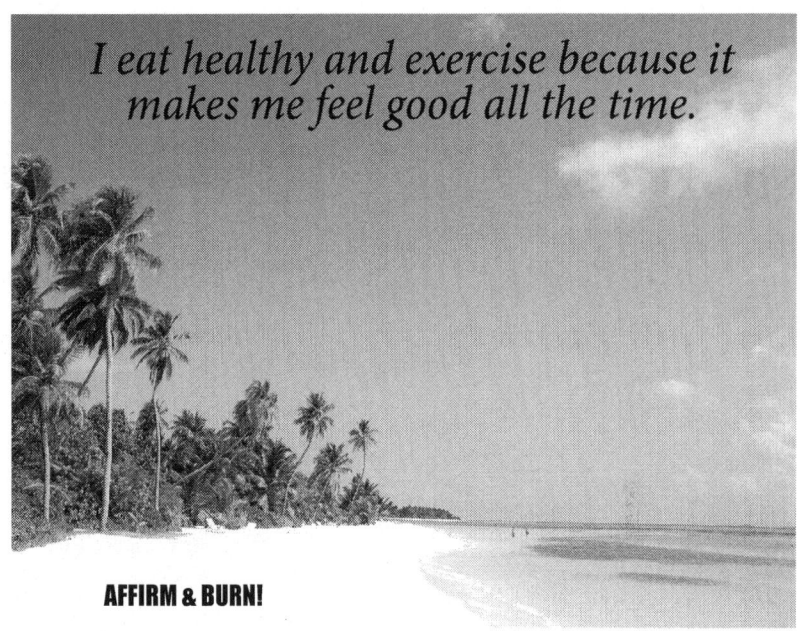

I eat healthy and exercise because it makes me feel good all the time.

AFFIRM & BURN!

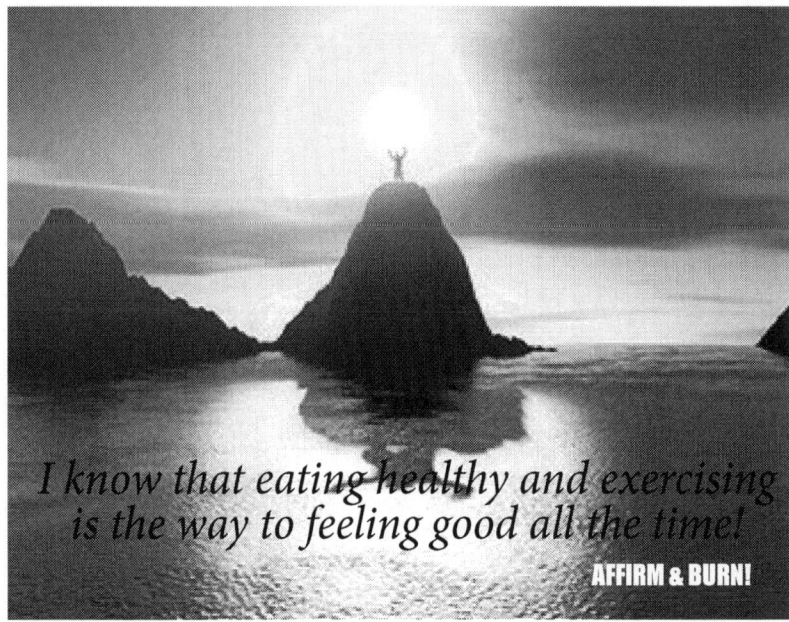

I know that eating healthy and exercising is the way to feeling good all the time!

AFFIRM & BURN!

*My body is filled
with love and light.
I feel lighter and
stronger every day.*

AFFIRM & BURN!

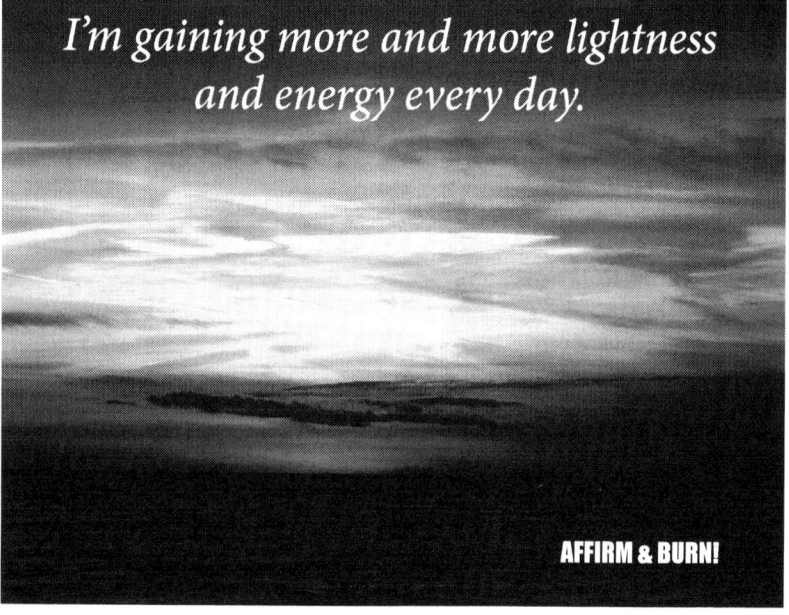

*I'm gaining more and more lightness
and energy every day.*

AFFIRM & BURN!

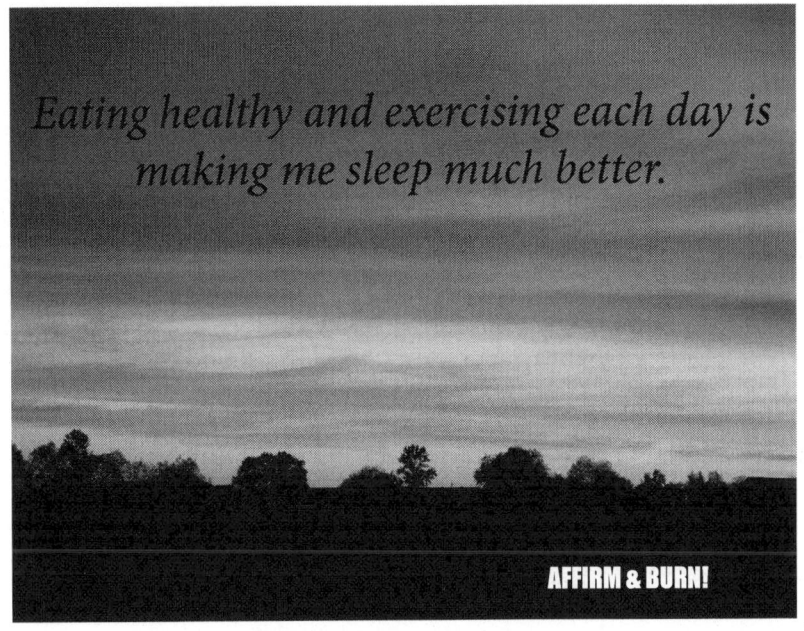

Eating healthy and exercising each day is making me sleep much better.

AFFIRM & BURN!

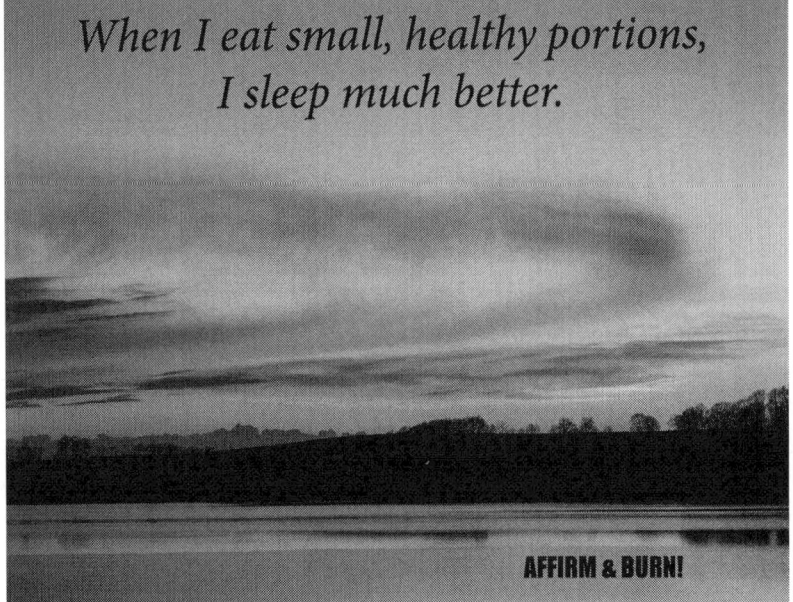

When I eat small, healthy portions, I sleep much better.

AFFIRM & BURN!

> *I sleep like a baby knowing I made great choices throughout the day.*
>
> **AFFIRM & BURN!**

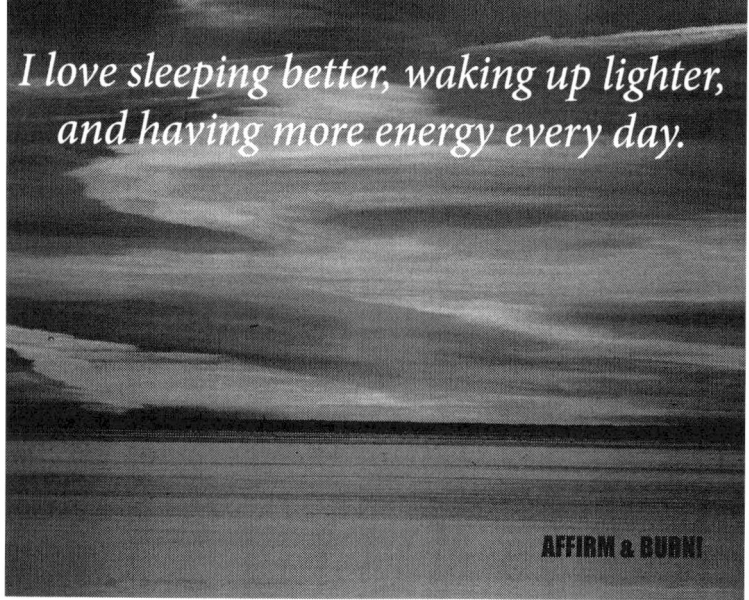

> *I love sleeping better, waking up lighter, and having more energy every day.*
>
> **AFFIRM & BURN!**

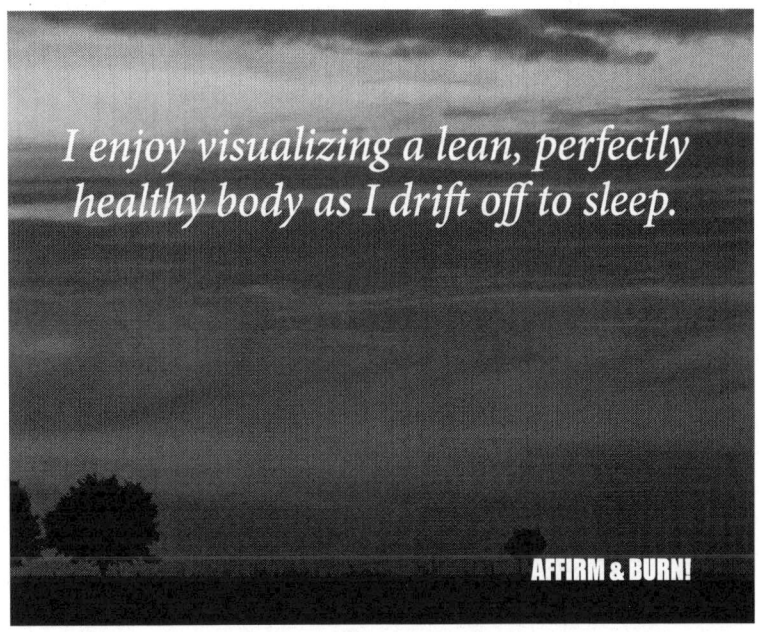

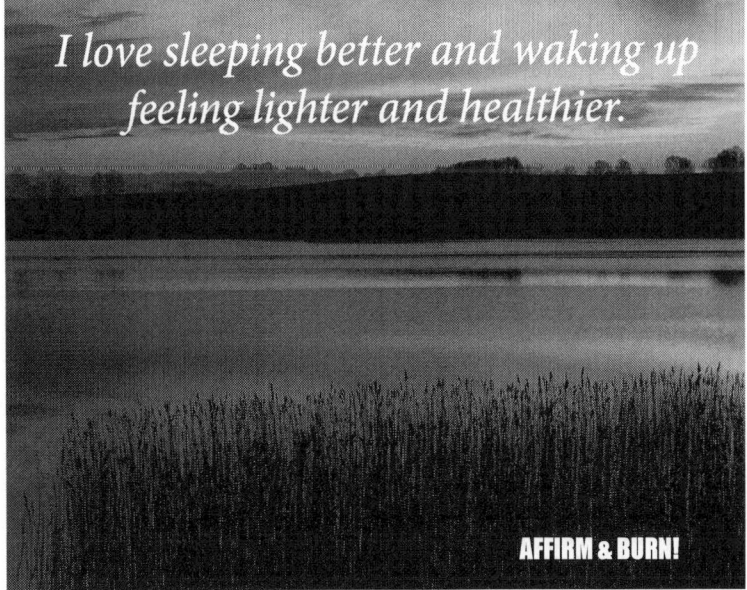

Post your favorite affirmations from the book onto the following photos.

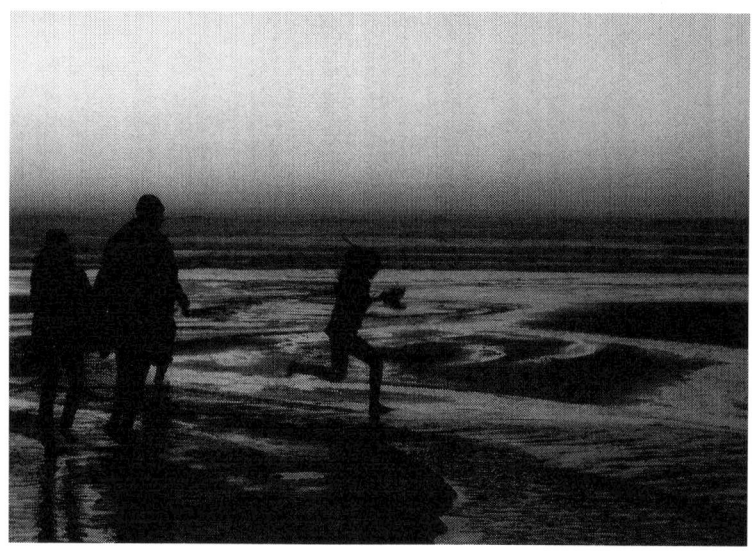

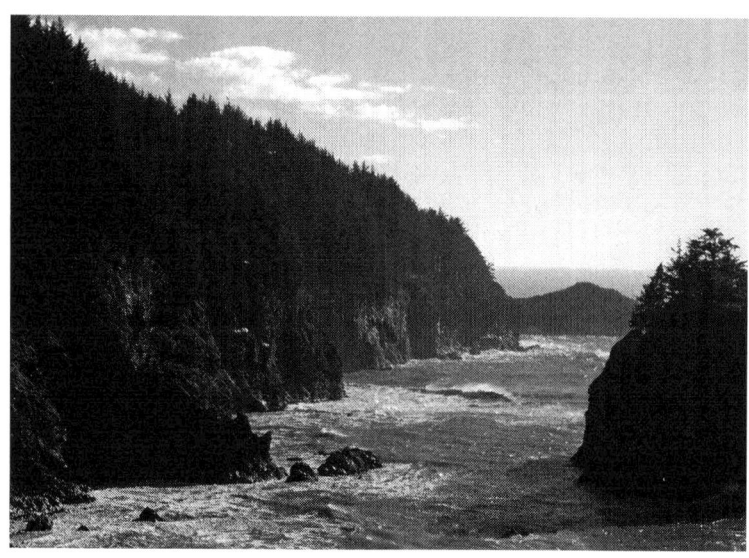

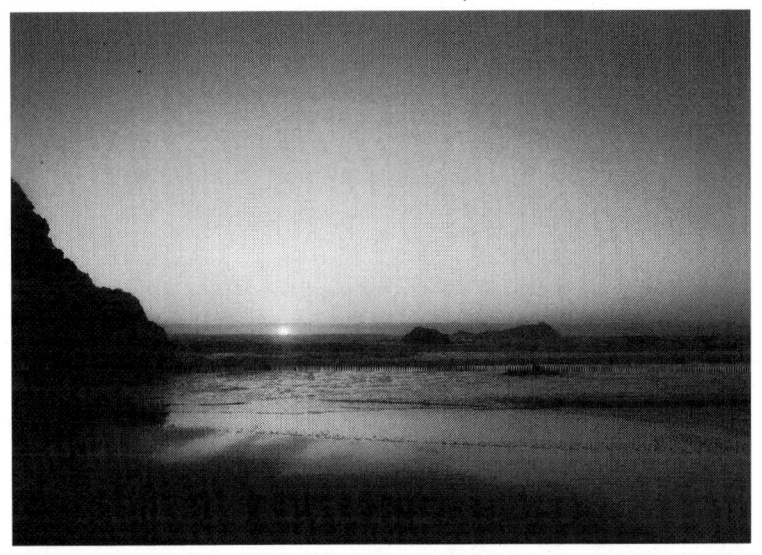

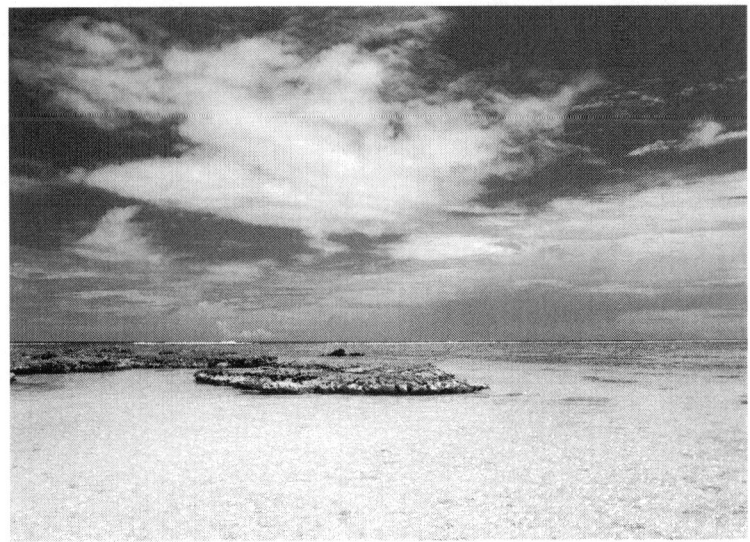

Affirm & Burn! is also available as an eBook on Amazon.